# OXFORD MEDICAL PUBLICATIONS

# *Medical imaging*

# Oxford Core Texts

CLINICAL DERMATOLOGY

PAEDIATRICS

ENDOCRINOLOGY

NEUROLOGY

PSYCHIATRY

MEDICAL IMAGING

# MEDICAL IMAGING

## Peter Scally

*Deputy Director of Radiology, Mater Hospital, Brisbane, Australia*
*Clinical Senior Lecturer, University of Queensland*

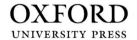

**OXFORD**
UNIVERSITY PRESS

# OXFORD
UNIVERSITY PRESS

Oxford University Press, Great Clarendon Street, Oxford OX2 6DP

Oxford  New York

Athens  Auckland  Bangkok  Bogota  Buenos Aires  Calcutta
Cape Town  Chennai  Dar es Salaam  Delhi  Florence  Hong Kong  Istanbul
Karachi  Kuala Lumpur  Madrid  Melbourne  Mexico City  Mumbai
Nairobi  Paris  São Paulo  Singapore  Taipei  Tokyo  Toronto  Warsaw

and associated companies in
Berlin Ibadan

Oxford is a trade mark of Oxford University Press

Published in the United States
by Oxford University Press, Inc., New York

A catalogue record for this book is available from the British Library

Library of Congress Cataloging in Publication Data
Scally, Peter.
Medical imaging/Peter Scally.
(Oxford core texts)
Includes bibliographical references and index.
ISBN 0 19 263056 3 (Pbk)
1. Diagnostic imaging.  I. Title.  II. Series.
[DNLM: 1. Diagnostic Imaging handbooks.  WN 39 S282m  1999]
RC78.7.D53S32  1999      616.07′54–dc21      98-55265

ISBN 0 19 263056 3

Typeset by
EXPO Holdings, Malaysia

Printed in China

To Catherine, Jason, and Elodie
While writing this book I have tried to keep my mind on what is important

When 500 students and clinicians were asked what they wanted from a radiology textbook, the replies indicated an emphasis on a system for reading X-rays, normal appearances, the appearances of common diseases, and planning an imaging strategy. Less important was information about contrast media, safety, and how images are produced. The book needed to be around 250 pages, A4 or pocket-book size, and inexpensive. These constraints have been adhered to. There is only so much time and effort that can be allocated to learning radiology. If a second edition of this book comes out it will have the same number of pages. The course is not getting any longer; why should the textbooks. If new information is added, something less important must be dropped.

Give an adult a computer game, a leisure activity, and watch the learning technique. The game is loaded and started. At times of need, the instructions are consulted. This book follows a similar path. Some skills in reading common films come first, followed by advice as to whether that was the correct film to request in the first place, and then an overview of what imaging achieves in the grand scheme. Some important information about safety and looking after people is also included.

The book is not an encyclopaedia of medical imaging. Additional learning must occur in lectures, tutorials, ward rounds, and in following the diagnosis and treatment of patients in clinical situations. The book aims to provide the basic knowledge that is essential, guided by simplicity and appropriateness, thus establishing a base on which future knowledge and complexity can be added. Some teachers may wish to cover certain areas in more detail. Students may eventually need more information about various facets of computed tomography (CT), or magnetic resonance imaging (MRI), or more about physics or barium studies. The Further Reading list indicates suitable reference texts.

The contents of this book have been decided on a 'need to know' basis:

- how to interpret basic radiographs;
- how to use imaging in solving clinical problems;
- information about safety and the role of radiology.

The three sections address these requirements, the structure of each section varying with its purpose.

Section 1 teaches how to look at common radiographs and to recognize the presence and nature of abnormalities.

The presence of an abnormality is detected by using a system for looking at the important areas and recognizing a deviation from normal. The normal is built up as a mental databank using a system of scrutiny that follows a perceptual flow. The abnormality is detected because it is too white, too black, or a distortion or displacement of a normal structure. This system applies whatever the image, be it an X-ray of the chest or ankle, or CT of the head. Once the abnormality is detected, it can be described in generic terms (e.g. consolidation, arthritis). A specific, pathological diagnosis may be appropriate if enough information is available. It is useful to link what is going on in the body with the images; an appreciation of why a disease process appears as it does: radiology reflecting pathology.

Section 1 is concerned with the acquisition and integration of knowledge (Marzano 1992). The knowledge is both declarative, in the form of facts, concepts, and principles to be learnt, and procedural, following formulae and strategies of thinking to arrive at a diagnosis. The invitation is there to associate, and compare and contrast the material, stimulating higher learning.

Sections 2 and 3 address a higher level of learning, concentrating on the meaningful use of knowledge and encompassing decision making, evaluating, problem solving, and clinical judgement. Section 2 discusses investigation of clinical problems and teaches a system of thinking that can be applied to resolve them. It encourages both clarity of thinking and using imaging wisely. Information about the different modalities and the appearances of important disorders is included. The more sophisticated studies are represented by examples, but these are restricted because non-radiologists do not usually report them.

Section 3 contains important information about the role of radiology, safety, care of the patient, and interventional radiology.

The material is kept simple in order that it may more easily become part of long-term memory and automatic response. Yet, woven through the text is an acknowledgement of the complexity of the subject and a reassurance that we are operating with less than perfect knowledge. It addresses uncertainty and decision making and teaches how to operate with limited information.

After reading this book once or twice certain skills should start to emerge:

- the ability to read normal and abnormal films;

- appreciation of radiology as the imaging of pathology;

- integration of radiology with the other clinical subjects;

- appropriate use of the resources in medical imaging—using the right test at the right time;

- clearer thinking using simple concepts, leading to less stress and more satisfaction.

The images presented have been carefully selected to cover common and important conditions. There are thousands more. Seeing them on a viewing box or monitor has two advantages over learning from books: one is that the radiographs are larger and have better resolution than photos; the other is that the human eye can detect many more grey scales when viewing images using transmitted light than with reflected light.

Each new unfamiliar appearance is a treasure to be followed up. This is adult, problem-based learning. The unfamiliar appearances become fewer with time.

*Brisbane*                                                                                                 P.S.
1999

# Acknowledgements

Dr Peter Bore who encouraged me to write and helped develop the ideas.

Drs Bob Fabiny, Colin Archibald, Robert Paterson, Warwick Carter, Simon Bowler, Jeremy Oates, Mark Ziervogel, Stephen Nutter, Graham Steele, Alexander Klestov, David Winkle, Peter Lavercombe, Kieran Frawley, Jack Harris, John Andersen, Roger Livsey, Anthony Lamont, Nick Tumman, Dan Petersen, John Tyrer, Peter Lennox, Ian Brown, Hemi Williams, Charles Mitchell, Hazel Tuck, Chris Pyke, Peter Hopkins, Des Soares, Scott Ingram, Peter Ross, Sue Jeavons, John Masel, Alex Phare, Clifford Bergman, Russell Park, Michael Sage, Paula Sivyer, Mark Burgin, Damayantha Seneviratne, Sutherland Mackechnie, John Ferguson, Michelle Nottage, Ian Skelly, and John Kerr who gave valuable advice and images.

Drs Ken Siddle, Jane Reasbeck, John Harper, Frances Archer and Mark Benson, who introduced me to radiology.

Charles Farrugia, Barry Martyn, Marnie Leighton, Adam Lack, Paul Duncan, Johann Koss, Sheila Aurisch, Rod van Twest, Jennifer Death, Scott Edie, Wendy Senior, Neville Cooper, Kris Kite, Lynne Holland, Michael Enright, Kerrin Kelly, Jeff Hassall, Deborah Quigg, Peter Butler, Richard Boytar, and Wendy Strugnell for their valuable advice, encouragement, and help with the production.

Many thanks to the talented and patient people at OUP.

# Contents

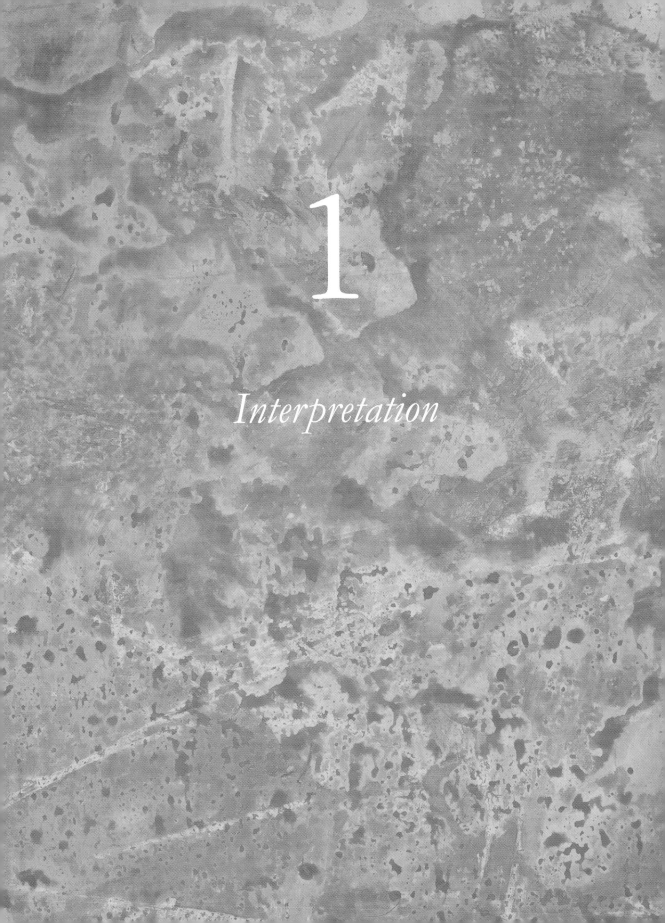

# 1

*Interpretation*

# *Interpretation*

Reading X-rays is like those quizzes in the Sunday newspaper where they say:
'Our artist made ten changes when copying the picture. Can you spot them?'

## SPOT THE DIFFERENCE

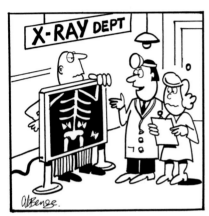 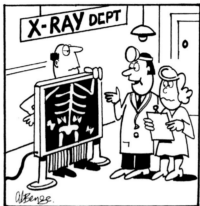

Except in radiology the original is not given for comparison, and no one says
how many changes there are. The original, or normal, radiograph for a person of
a certain age and sex is a mental image that must be developed. The best way to
build up this mental picture is to use a consistent system to examine radiographs. In this way, not only will abnormalities be detected, but much will be
learnt, even with a normal study.

The aim of this section is to teach:

- how to interpret basic radiographs—to do this a basic knowledge of anatomy
  and pathology is required;

- normal radiological anatomy;

- how to look at the radiographs;

  where to look, covering the important areas and emphasizing perceptual flow;

  what to look for when reading chest, abdominal, and skeletal radiographs—
  basically an abnormal density, abnormal radiolucency, or distortion or displacement of a normal structure: in other words something too white, too
  black, or distorted or out of place;

- what the abnormalities commonly mean and how the pathophysiology causes
  such appearances. Either the radiograph is called normal or an abnormality is
  detected. Describe the abnormality in generic terms or in specific terms if
  possible.

By the end of this section you should be able to approach the reading of an X-ray in a systematic fashion, to detect if there is an abnormality, to diagnose some common diseases, and to know when to seek assistance for those that are less clear.

An important consideration is that there is little benefit in interpreting images if the wrong ones are requested. Sections 2 and 3 give some guidance in clinical thinking and how to order the correct test.

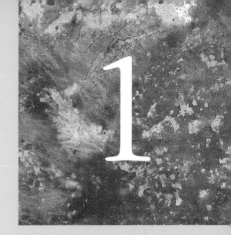

1

# Chest X-rays

Interpreting plain films, such as those of the chest, complements the other abilities of a clinician and adds understanding.

There are good reasons to start with acquiring the skill of reading chest X-rays (CXR): they are the most common radiographs; they may arrive without a radiologist's report; interpretation can be a life-or-death matter; and they are the most difficult single image to interpret. A systematic approach is needed for best results.

## Systematic approach

Try placing a chest X-ray upside down on the viewing box. All the information is there but it is difficult to interpret because it is not presented in the usual way; your perception is disorientated. Let us therefore accept that having a system for viewing images will make life easier.

The systematic approach has many benefits: it minimizes the chance of missing an abnormality; enables detection of a second or related lesion; makes complex images easier to read with practice; and builds up a mental databank of what is normal. It is not possible to call a film abnormal if the normal appearance is not known.

Read this chapter while sitting *directly* in front of a viewing box with a CXR displayed. Optimize the viewing conditions by turning off adjacent lights.

For chest X-rays, devise a system for yourself that covers the following fields:

(1) the documentary evidence of name and age;

(2) technical factors;

(3) areas of interest:

  (a) lungs

  (b) pleura

  (c) mediastinum and heart

  (d) hila

  (e) bones

  (f) soft tissues.

> ### Hint
> It can be difficult to see details of X-rays when they are printed in a book. With reflected light, fewer shades of grey can be seen compared with viewing an X-ray on a viewing box with transmitted light or on a good monitor.

Link each feature to the following one so that a perceptual flow develops. Do not try to cover two areas such as the lungs and bones at once. This is a high-risk strategy, making it easier to miss something. It would be like trying to look up two names in the phone book—it's quicker to do one at a time.

Each of the six areas of interest is described in the following pages. Remember that an abnormality can only be one of three things:

(1) an opacity

(2) a radiolucency

(3) a distortion or displacement of a normal structure.

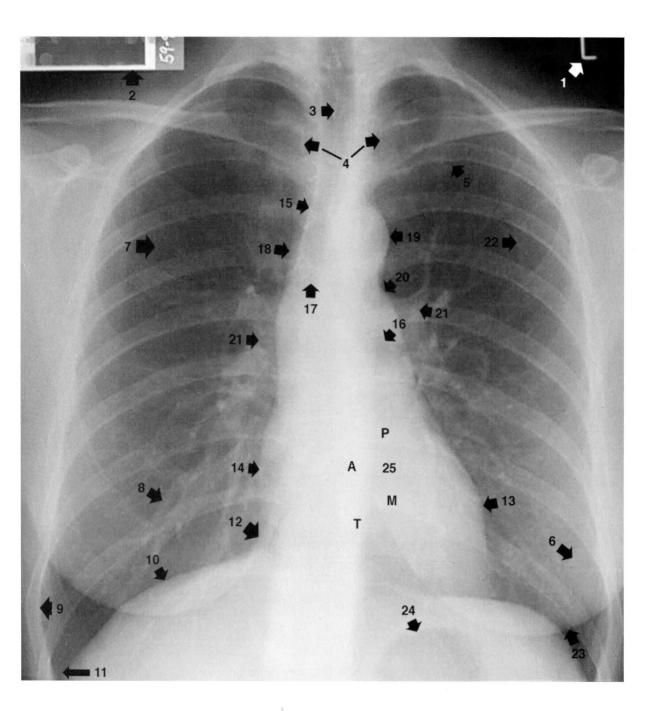

Examples of these three groups of abnormalities will be presented, followed by a section on how to interpret common pathology in the chest and an introduction to chest computed tomography (CT).

The following description is *one* approach to reading a chest X-ray, having good perceptual flow as well as emphasizing the important structures first. Your

**Fig.** 1.1 Normal CXR.

Annotations:

(1) side marker—the CXR and most other plain films are viewed as if the patient is facing you;

(2) name—usually in *this position* in a PA film because it is fixed by the design of the cassette—if the name is back to front, it is because the radiographer printed it that way;

(3) thoracic spinous process;

(4) ends of the clavicles—equidistant from the spinous processes (to check for rotation to the right or left) and at the level of T4 (to check for rotation forward or backward), if the patient is leaning to one side it is obvious and usually because they are unwell;

(5) first rib—when counting the ribs start with the anterior end of the first;

(6) seventh rib—with normal lung volumes the hemidiaphragm is at the level of the 5th–7th ribs anteriorly;

(7) lung density—varies with exposure factors and disease;

(8) pulmonary marking, vessels, and bronchi—the peripheral markings are the arteries and veins;

(9) pleura—this is where the pleura is, but it is usually only visible when abnormal—normal pleura, two layers of visceral pleura, is visible as the fissures but only when seen end-on;

(10) hemidiaphragm—there is only one diaphragm, but the two sides can work independently so it is useful to refer to the right and left hemidiaphragms;

(11) costophrenic angle;

(12) cardiophrenic angle;

(13) part of the left ventricle forms the left heart border;

(14) part of the right atrium forms the right heart border—the left atrium is around the back and part of its wall provides the posterior border of the heart in the lateral film (correlate this with the CT of the heart chambers, later in this chapter);

(15) trachea—normally deviated to the right by the arch of the aorta;

(16) left main bronchus;

(17) carina—the bifurcation of the trachea;

(18) paratracheal tissues, vessels;

(19) aortic arch—also called the aortic knuckle;

(20) pulmonary artery (correlate this with the CT appearance);

(21) hila—the density is caused by the pulmonary artery and superior pulmonary vein;

(22) edge of the scapula;

(23) breast outline;

(24) stomach bubble;

(25) heart valves.

own method may be different. No problem there. Just remember the rules: do it the same way each time; develop a comfortable perceptual flow; and cover the important areas.

## Start with the documentary evidence

Check the name, age, and whether the film is PA (posteroanterior, the X-ray beam coming from behind, with the cassette anterior to the patient) or AP (anteroposterior). The name-tag is usually in the top-left corner as you face the film in a PA projection (top-right for AP). Some hospitals may use the reverse orientation. Chest films are done PA if possible in order to assess the heart size. Patients examined with portable equipment usually have an AP film, as they are lying supine or sitting in bed.

A supine film has implications. One is that it is an AP film and the heart size will be exaggerated. The other implications are related to gravity:

• Pleural fluid will layer posteriorly and give an increased density to the hemithorax.

- A pneumothorax will lie anteriorly and will be difficult to detect.
- The diaphragm will be higher and reduce the lung volumes.
- Prominence of the upper zone vessels is normal and does not reflect left heart failure as it often does in an erect radiograph.

## Technical factors

- Check the side marker.
- Rotation is best assessed by looking at the medial ends of the clavicles. They should be equidistant from the thoracic spinous processes which mark the midline, and at about the level of T4 in a PA film. Rotation in any one of the three planes can cause difficulties with densities or appearances. An example would be apparent widening of the mediastinum when the patient is rotated to the right or left.
- With a normal penetration/exposure of the film, the upper half of the thoracic spine should be distinguishable.

This may seem tedious but it can be assessed at a glance with a little practice. With experience always check the name and then go to the six areas of interest. Any technical problems will become obvious.

## Areas of interest

### Lungs

This is where most of the pathology is shown, so it is a good place to start. Look at the lung *volumes*. The hemidiaphragms should be at the level of the fifth to seventh rib anteriorly or the tenth rib posteriorly. It is easier to count anterior ribs; start with the first.

## What to look for (lung volumes)

### Distortion of a structure

### Small lungs

(a) bilaterally:
- supine position
- suboptimal inspiration
- obesity
- fibrotic lungs
- fluid-filled lungs from cardiac failure
- causes below the diaphragm, such as late pregnancy or distended bowel

(b) unilaterally:
- something in the lung (collapse, fibrosis)

## What to look for (lung volumes) (continued)

- something in the wall of the hemithorax, including the chest wall, the mediastinum, and hemidiaphragm (pain of a rib fracture, phrenic nerve palsy, cerebrovascular accident (CVA) paralysing the chest wall and diaphragm, mesothelioma)
- something outside the wall (contralateral tension pneumothorax pushing the mediastinum across, subphrenic abscess elevating the hemidiaphragm)

### Overexpanded lungs

- chronic airflow obstruction such as emphysema, asthma. (See HINT.)

### A large hemithorax can be caused by:

- tension pneumothorax

Is each hemithorax of normal *radiolucency*? (footnote 1) If not, which is the abnormal side? Judging normal density is difficult for the novice, but becomes easier with practice.

Next, look for any abnormal *opacity*. Start at the base of the right lung and examine it as far as the apex. Jump to the apex of the left lung and examine it down to the base.

---

1 Radiolucent means something which allows the X-ray photons to pass with little deflection or absorption (lucent = shining or transparent). Gas or air is most radiolucent because of the low density. Soft tissues of the body are relatively radiolucent because they are composed of atoms that have low atomic numbers. The most common atoms in the body are hydrogen (atomic number of 1), oxygen (atomic number of 8), and carbon (atomic number of 6). X-rays that pass through will expose the film—either directly or by causing light to be emitted from the intensifying screens—and make the film black when developed.

An opacity means something that stops the X-rays and will therefore appear white. Bones contain calcium (atomic number of 20), an atom with 20 electrons and better X-ray stopping power.

Same system for white and black in CT.

In ultrasound white means something that sends back an echo, such as a calculus or an interface with gas, and is called echogenic or hyperechoic. Hypoechoic substances (black) are fluids with little or no particulate matter.

In radionuclear scans the active sites of accumulation of the isotope give out gamma rays that can be detected by a gamma camera. On the resultant image these sites will appear black (hot spots or areas of increased activity). Gamma rays are the same as X-rays, being photons with similar energies.

White in magnetic resonance imaging (MRI) means high signal intensity. The same structure can have a high signal in one sequence and a low signal in another. It gets a bit complicated. Get friendly with terms like signal void (black), high signal (white), and low signal and people will think you know what you are talking about.

### Hint

With obstruction of airflow one might expect to see small lungs. The lungs are, however, enlarged. This seems counter-intuitive, but the explanation goes as follows: in both asthma and emphysema the lumen of the small airways is narrowed: in asthma from thickened walls and mucus in the lumen, in emphysema from loss of alveolar walls. The alveolar walls hold the bronchioles open by radial traction.

Two effects contribute to big lungs:

1. People with asthma and emphysema like to keep their lung volumes big (large residual volume). More radial traction. It keeps the airways open.

2. In expiration the airways have slightly smaller diameters and hence more resistance to flow. Flow is proportional to the *fourth* power of the diameter. Air gets in but has trouble getting out: a partial ball-valve effect.

Obstructive lung disease often causes big lungs, while restrictive lung disease gives small lungs.

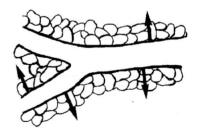

**Fig. 1.2** Radial traction on a bronchiole. As the chest expands the elasticity of the alveolar walls pulls on the bronchiole walls to increase the diameter of the airways.

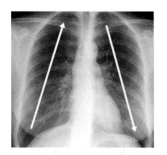

**Fig.** 1.3 Looking at the lungs.

## Hint

Looking at a normal lung the only feature (opacity) that can always be seen is the vasculature, both veins and arteries. In the lung periphery these cannot be distinguished one from the other. The vessels should spread out from the hila and be perceivable for about 80% of the distance to the chest wall. If lung markings are visible further than this it could be because of underpenetration. In such a case check that the upper few vertebrae of the thorax can be seen. If so, exposure is adequate and the cause of the increased markings is thickened bronchial walls, interstitial disease, or, in children, increased blood flow in the lungs from a left to right shunt.

Distortion of the distribution of the vessels is abnormal.

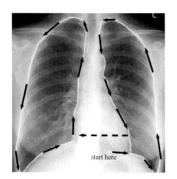

**Fig.** 1.4 Looking at the pleura.

# What to look for (radiolucency)

### Opaque hemithorax (relatively white):

- small lung
- rotation of the patient
- pleural effusion in the supine position

### Radiolucent hemithorax (relatively black):

- technical fault (patient is rotated)
- something in the lung (pulmonary embolus by arresting the blood flow, emphysema by destruction of lung parenchyma distal to the terminal bronchioles)
- pleural (pneumothorax)
- chest wall (mastectomy)

### Bilateral radiolucent hemithorax:

- asthma, emphysema, or bronchiolitis in children

# What to look for (abnormal opacity)

### Opacity: in the lung

- consolidation
- collapse
- nodules from 1 mm to 3 cm in size
- nodules larger than 3 cm are called masses
- lines which are straight or curvilinear

### Pleura

Pleura covers the lungs. The best place to look for pleural disease is in profile, i.e. around the lung margins. This technique has the advantage of making sure the lung peripheries are seen.

Start at the left cardiophrenic angle and move along the hemidiaphragm to the left costophrenic angle. Follow the border of the lung up to the apex and then down the mediastinal edge, noting the aortic arch, pulmonary artery, and left heart border.

Move across to the right cardiophrenic angle.

Follow the mediastinal edge of the right heart border, ascending aorta, and brachiocephalic vessels to the apex and down the lateral wall to the costophrenic angle and back across the hemidiaphragm to the right cardiophrenic angle.

# What to look for (pleura)

*Opacities:*

- an effusion
- plaques or thickening
- mass lesion

*Distortion:*

- Loss of clarity of the pleural edge—particularly of the left hemidiaphragm and of the left and right heart borders—is called the silhouette sign. The silhouette sign is positive when there is loss of the silhouette. It indicates adjacent lung disease such as consolidation or collapse, or a pleural effusion.

*Displacement:*

- Displacement of the pleura occurs with a pneumothorax or pleural effusion.

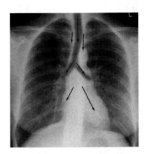

Fig. 1.5 Looking at the mediastinum.

## Mediastinum and heart

Start at the top. Check the trachea, right and left main bronchi, right and left paratracheal spaces, aortic arch, pulmonary artery, and the heart. The density of the right side of the heart should be the same as that of the left side. Also look at the vertebral bodies. Remember that the thoracic inlet is oblique. Anteriorly, anything above the clavicles is in the neck. Posteriorly (in a PA CXR) the thorax is higher, up to the level of the T1 vertebra.

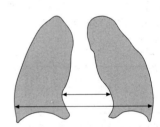

Fig. 1.6 How to measure the cardiothoracic ratio.

# What to look for (mediastinum)

*Opacity:*

- masses in the mediastinum (goitre, tortuous brachiocephalic (innominate) artery, lymph nodes, tumours, calcification). If the left side of the heart appears abnormally opaque, it usually means left lower lobe consolidation and/or collapse. Look for an accompanying positive silhouette sign, loss of clarity of the left hemidiaphragm.

*Radiolucency:*

- pneumomediastinum. Gas does not reach the mediastinum from a pneumothorax. It comes from a penetrating injury, or from rupture of the trachea or more distal airways, or of the oesophagus.

*Distortion or displacement:*

- shift of the mediastinum. Is it being pushed or pulled?
- enlarged heart. In a PA film the heart should be no broader than 50% of the widest internal diameter of the chest, i.e. a cardiothoracic ratio (CTR) of <50%, or be no greater in width than 15.5 cm in adults. In the supine (AP)

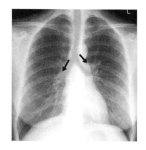

Fig. 1.7 Looking at the hila.

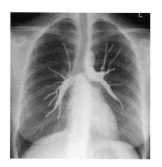

Fig. 1.8 Diagram of the hila.

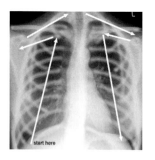

Fig. 1.9 Looking at the bones.

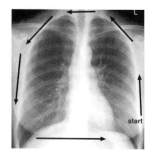

Fig. 1.10 Looking at the soft tissues.

## What to look for (mediastinum) (continued)

CXR the heart is considered enlarged if the left heart border abuts the lateral chest wall, or if the CTR is greater than 60%, or the cardiac size is >19 cm (Van der Jagt and Smits 1992). Enlargement occurs with ischaemic heart disease, valvular heart disease, pericardial effusion, pericardial fat in obesity, and cardiomyopathy. The heart size can vary by 1 cm between systole and diastole. Comparison with a previous size is more useful than a single reading. An echocardiogram is the best way to tell which chamber is enlarged, if that is important.

- distorted shape of the heart—congenital heart disease, valvular heart disease.

### The hila

Look carefully. Each hilum is the result of the density of the pulmonary artery and the *superior* pulmonary vein. The main bronchus is there but does not add much to the density. The *inferior* pulmonary vein enters the left atrium well below the hilum.

The left hilum is 1 cm higher than that on the right because the left pulmonary artery arches up and over the left main bronchus.

The hila become easier to interpret with practice.

## What to look for (hila)

### Opacity:

- One hilum bigger or more dense than the other:

  carcinoma;

  lymph node enlargement caused by lymphoma, metastatic tumour, infection, or sarcoidosis;

  large pulmonary arteries due to pulmonary arterial hypertension, usually secondary to chronic lung disease such as emphysema (but sometimes it is a primary disorder or is caused by thromboembolic disease).

### Distortion:

- The hila may pulled up or down by fibrosis or collapse of the lung.

### Bones

Start at the right lower ribs. Check each rib up to the first, look at the right shoulder girdle, the spine, the left shoulder girdle, and the left ribs.

### Soft tissues

Scan the left breast shadow and chest wall, soft tissues of the neck, and then look down the right chest wall and right breast tissue ending with a glance below the diaphragm.

## What to look for (bones)

*Opacity:*

- secondary of prostate or breast cancer
- healing fracture

*Radiolucency:*

- rib fracture
- secondary deposit

## What to look for (soft tissues)

*Opacity:*

- neck masses

*Radiolucency:*

- pneumoperitoneum
- subcutaneous emphysema
- mastectomy

### Tips and tricks

If there are two or more chest X-rays always place them in chronological order from left to right. There are enough variables to consider without having to remember which film came first.

## The lateral film

Some centres do not use the lateral CXR routinely because the radiation dose is five times that of the PA exposure. It is a useful view for confirming the position of lesions, particularly nodules, to see if they are in the lung.

Check four areas:

(1) *the retrosternal space* where the two lungs meet anterior to the ascending aorta and the remains of the thymus;

## What to look for (retrosternal space)

*Opacity:*

- enlarged right ventricle
- anterior mediastinal mass such as a thymoma, thyroid mass or goitre, teratoma, or terrible lymphoma (4 Ts)

*Radiolucency:*

- hyperinflated lungs

(2) *the subcarinal region*;

## What to look for (subcarinal region)

### Opacity:

- enlarged nodes

(3) *the vertebral bodies*. Normally the thoracic vertebral bodies appear increasingly more radiolucent (increasingly black) from superior to inferior until the hemidiaphragms are reached at about the level of the body of T11. If the vertebral bodies appear unduly opaque it is usually because of a superimposed pleural effusion, consolidation, or bronchial wall thickening.

## What to look for (vertebral bodies)

### Opacity:

- density caused by disease in the lung bases
- collapsed vertebra
- dense vertebral body of Paget's disease or malignancy

### Distortion:

- collapsed vertebra

(4) *the posterior costophrenic angle*. Consolidation or a pleural effusion can cause loss of the silhouette of the adjacent hemidiaphragm, although it is sometimes difficult to say whether it is on the right or left. Look for the stomach gas bubble under the left hemidiaphragm. The right hemidiaphragm extends further forward than the left.

## What to look for (posterior costophrenic angle)

### Opacity:

- pleural effusion
- consolidation
- Bochdalek hernia (a congenital defect of the diaphragm, containing retroperitoneal fat or part of the kidney)

There are other views of the chest apart from the PA and lateral projections. To cover them here would add unnecessary complexity and would be against the philosophy and limitations of this book. The other projections will become apparent when you ask the question: 'What do I need to know?' See Section 2. Enlargement of cardiac chambers is assessed with ultrasound.

Before continuing, be sure to read the Preface.

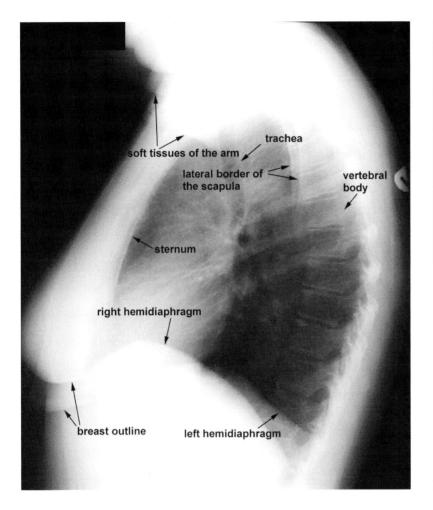

soft tissues of the arm

trachea

lateral border of
the scapula

vertebral
body

sternum

right hemidiaphragm

breast outline

left hemidiaphragm

**Fig.** 1.12 Lateral CXR.

## Correlation of lung pathology and the chest X-ray appearances

Detection of the abnormality is the first hurdle to overcome. The information you now have is an opacity, radiolucency, or distortion or displacement of a normal structure. This needs to be converted to an estimate of the underlying pathology.

**Note:**

1. Care is needed because many diseases can have similar appearances on a chest X-ray.

2. It may only be possible to make a generic diagnosis, such as consolidation. However, the clinical features may supply additional information to allow a specific diagnosis: pneumonia, pulmonary oedema, or haemorrhage—old films will tell you if it is acute or chronic. The distribution will indicate if it is diffuse or localized. A lung biopsy may be needed to determine the aetiology, and even then it can be uncertain. Who said medicine was easy?

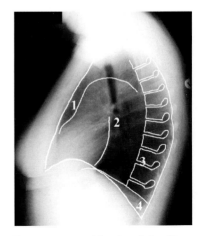

**Fig.** 1.11 Perceptual flow, lateral chest X-ray.

3. It is unwise to diagnose with inadequate information. Knowing when there is enough data to confirm that a disease is present is a clinical skill that comes with good learning techniques and experience.

Before looking at the lung pathologies, let us digress to explain one important concept, that radiology is the imaging of pathology. Chest X-rays are a two-dimensional, black and white representation of normal structures and pathology. Knowledge of normal appearances and of macroscopic pathology is essential. Unfortunately, clarity of thinking about pathology is often suboptimal. If students are asked 'What is the pathological definition of bronchiectasis', they often reply 'Irreversible dilatation of the bronchial tree' but leave out the important rider '…caused by or accompanied by chronic, necrotizing infection'. Those who take the time to learn the basis of each disease in one sentence find that much of the complexity of medicine disappears. A good definition will tell you what the radiological findings should be. Take the example of bronchiectasis. The CXR will show dilated bronchi with thickened walls seen as circles when end-on or as parallel lines when seen side-on. The second part of the definition implies that destructive infection can erode the walls to form abscesses in the parenchyma giving small opacities and an increase in the interstitial markings. These infections heal with scarring. This scarring or fibrosis involves contraction, as it does in other parts of the body, and approximation of the dilated bronchi. Gravity determines that the pathology is usually at the lung bases. Plain films may show these changes but CT demonstrates them better. The treatment is obvious from the definition—drainage and physical therapy, antibiotics, and perhaps surgery to remove a scarred and shrunken lobe.

The abnormalities in the CXR can be grouped as:

* opacities

* radiolucencies

* distortion or displacement of a normal structure.

## Opacities

(1) Large

* consolidation

* collapse

* pleural fluid

(2) Nodules and masses

(3) Linear opacities can be lines that are straight, curvilinear, or circular, acute or chronic, and localized or diffuse.

### Large opacities in the thorax
#### Consolidation

Consolidation, also known as 'air-space (acinar) disease' or 'alveolar opacity', is seen on an X-ray when a substance, usually fluid, fills the alveolar air spaces but not the airways (bronchial tree). The fluid can be a *transudate* of pulmonary oedema, *pus* of infection/pneumonia or *blood* from trauma or bleeding from a tumour, an area of infection, or vasculitis.

Consolidation is an example of how the lung is a highly specialized organ and can only respond to injuries in a limited number of ways. The reactions to inflammation and left heart failure are similar, with fluid entering the interstitial tissues from the capillaries—through loosening of the endothelial bonds in one case or increased hydrostatic pressure in the other. More severe disease will see the fluid pass between the pneumocytes and enter the alveolar air spaces, giving a picture of consolidation. Sometimes the fluid of consolidation is inhaled directly, as occurs with drowning or bleeding from the bronchial tree.

The radiographic appearance of consolidation, of this fluid filling the alveolar air spaces, logically follows. It is poorly defined, has a tendency to confluence (running together), is limited by the fissures, is usually not associated with any change in volume, and contains an air-bronchogram (fluid fills the segment of the lung but the branching, bronchial tree is visible because it contains air; i.e. fluid fills the air spaces but not the airways).

Once the generic diagnosis of consolidation is made, the specific diagnosis can be deduced, by looking at its distribution and by using additional information obtained from the history and examination.

## Collapse

Partial or complete collapse of one or more bronchopulmonary segments can lead to characteristic appearances, although the distortion produced by the collapse is sometimes confusing. Atelectasis is a small area of collapse. The causes of collapse/atelectasis are:

- relaxation (a result of the elasticity) of the lung parenchyma as occurs with a pneumothorax or pleural effusion;
- obstruction of a bronchus/bronchiole;
- fibrosis which contracts the lung with a consequent loss of volume.

Obstruction of a bronchus can be luminal, mural, or extramural. Luminal causes include: mucus plugs; a foreign body; or perhaps an endotracheal tube in the right main bronchus, obstructing the left. Neoplasms are the main mural cause. Occasionally tumours and large lymph nodes can compress the bronchus from outside the wall.

However, collapse is not the only consequence of bronchial obstruction. Complete or partial obstruction may lead to a variety of appearances:

- Collapse.
- Obstructive emphysema where the airway obstruction is complete during expiration. With inspiration, the diameter of the bronchus increases because of pull on the wall by the lung septae and alveolar walls, and more air fills the distal, distended air spaces. It establishes a one-way valve effect and occurs with inhaled foreign bodies. The same principle applies more diffusely in obstructive airways disease, a form of generalized air trapping.
- Obstructive pneumonitis which is usually caused by a neoplasm. The distal bronchial tree and alveoli fill with secretions. There is no loss of volume.
- Pneumonia.
- Bronchiectasis.

**Hint**

Two rules of thumb are:

1. If the consolidation is bilaterally symmetrical it is often due to left heart failure.

2. When focal consolidation is present consider pulmonary infarction and haemorrhage from an embolus as an alternative to pneumonia.

Collapse is demonstrated by an opacity and loss of volume. This shrinkage is shown by a small hemithorax with deviation of the mediastinum, elevation of the hemidiaphragm, hilar shift, and approximation of the ribs. Interestingly, the hemithorax may actually be more radiolucent because of the expansion of the remainder of the lung to fill the space.

### Pleural fluid

Fluid in the pleural space can be detected once there is more than 100 ml present. In the erect film it is seen in the lateral or posterior costophrenic angles as a meniscus that curves up the chest wall. Sometimes the fluid layers between the lung and diaphragm to give a subpulmonic effusion and apparent elevation of the hemidiaphragm. A lateral decubitus film or ultrasound will confirm this finding. A fluid level will be seen in the pleural space under two conditions:

(1) both fluid and air are present;

(2) the X-ray beam is horizontal.

Pleural effusions are often the result of pulmonary oedema, either of cardiogenic or non-cardiogenic origin, and will often be bilateral. Cardiogenic pulmonary oedema is common and is usually a result of left heart failure, or, less commonly, mitral valve disease. Non-cardiogenic examples are fluid overload with renal failure, drug reaction, and the acute respiratory distress syndrome (ARDS). Pleural effusions also occur unilaterally with adjacent lung disease such as: infection, infarction, tumour and with trauma, surgery, subphrenic inflammation, and immunological diseases, for example rheumatoid arthritis. The fluid can be a transudate or exudate, haemorrhagic or chylous (lymph fluid). An empyema is pus in the pleural cavity.

### Nodules and masses

Spherical densities are more appropriately called nodules rather than coin lesions because they are three-dimensional. They range in size from 1 mm to many centimetres, but when larger than 3 cm they are called masses.

Hundreds of 1 mm nodules imply the presence of miliary tuberculosis until proven otherwise. Miliary means like millet seeds. They are small.

Solitary or multiple nodules in the lungs are usually neoplastic or infective, but the differential diagnosis includes at least 20 other items (footnote 2).

---

2  Causes of pulmonary nodules:

- granulomas: tuberculoma, histoplasmoma
- malignant neoplasms: primary and secondary
- benign neoplasms: adenoma, hamartoma
- infections: hydatid
- vascular: arteriovenous malformation, haematoma

More important than what they could be is what they are. If presented with a CXR with a 10-mm nodule in the right mid-zone, your thinking and report to a medical colleague should go something like this: 'A 10-mm nodule is present in the right mid-zone and its location is confirmed in the lateral film. There is no other abnormality in the lungs, mediastinum, or ribs. Both breast shadows are present. Comparison with old films is desirable in the first instance. If it has appeared or grown in the last two years, it requires further work-up. Correlation with the history and clinical findings such as a history of cancer, travel, cough or fever, and the white cell count and sputum analysis may be useful. A CT would reveal any other nodules and the presence of enlarged mediastinal nodes. Diagnostic material may be obtained by bronchoscopy or fine-needle aspiration.'

*Linear markings are straight, curved, or circular*

(1) *Straight*

    (a) acute (hours to days)

        • localized

        • diffuse

    (b) chronic (weeks, months, or years)

        • localized

        • diffuse

(2) *Curvilinear*

(3) *Circular*

*Straight* linear markings mean *interstitial* disease, atelectasis, or scarring. Compare that with consolidation which means *air-space* disease. Air spaces are the alveolar sacs and alveoli.

The interstitium is the tissue that lies between the basement membranes of the capillaries and of the pneumocytes, under the pleura and around the vessels. It is essentially fluid with a few cells. The lung *parenchyma* is the interstitium plus the alveolar walls, vessels, bronchi, lymphatics, and nodes.

The appearances of lung parenchyma diseases are varied:

• Disease of the alveolar walls is pneumonitis. Later, the alveolar spaces may fill with fluid, producing air-space disease.

• Diseases of the vessels are vasculitis and thromboembolism and produce bleeding or infarction.

• Diseases of the bronchi are those of inflammation (bronchitis and asthma), obstruction, and tumours.

• Diseases of the lymphatics and nodes are usually infection, but those seen on a CXR are more often tumours. Sometimes cells and fluid block the lymphatics, causing the linear markings and air-space disease of lymphangitis carcinomatosa.

• Diseases of the interstitium need more description.

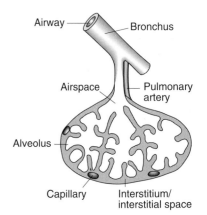

**Fig. 1.13** The lung interstitium.

Interstitial disease consists of fluid and usually inflammatory cells that escape from the capillaries into the surrounding interstitium. The appearances are essentially of linear densities and small nodules. One or the other may predominate.

The nodules are accumulations of cells such as interstitial cells, mast cells, fibroblasts, and chronic inflammatory cells (lymphocytes and macrophages).

The interstitial fluid will give CXR findings of: linear markings; peribronchial thickening; loss of clarity of the vessel walls; and a slight increase in lung opacity because of thickening of the interstitium. Lung compliance is decreased so the volumes may be small. Lines are seen because it is only the septa aligned with the X-ray beam that absorb or deflect enough photons to be visible. The lines may criss-cross to give a web or net appearance, called a reticular (footnote 3) pattern. If the lines are too thin and beyond the resolution of the CXR or CT it gives a hazy appearance called a ground-glass pattern.

Radiological signs of interstitial disease are therefore reticular, nodular, reticulonodular opacities, or a ground-glass appearance. End-stage disease has a honeycomb appearance due to lung destruction and its replacement with thick, fibrous septa and cyst formation.

The classification of interstitial lung disease is:

*acute*

- localized
- diffuse

*chronic*

- localized
- diffuse

1. Acute interstitial disease

   *Localized* changes occur with infections in the early phase such as with mycoplasma, pneumocystis, and viral pneumonias. The inflammatory fluid is seen as a vague increase in lung markings and a few lines.

   *Diffuse*, acute interstitial disease indicates pulmonary oedema, of cardiogenic or non-cardiogenic aetiology. Left heart failure is the most common source, but always remember infection and the other non-cardiogenic causes in the differential diagnosis. Understanding the disease will make the radiology simple. Consider cardiac failure. Atherosclerosis causes coronary artery disease—which causes myocardial ischaemia—which in turn gives left heart failure. The end-diastolic pressure in the left ventricle increases and so must the left atrial pressure. This leads to pulmonary *venous* hypertension, shown initially as upper zone vascular redistribution. As the failure worsens, the hydrostatic pressure causes fluid to flow into the interstitial space. This gives an appearance of straight lines up to 2 cm in length and 1 mm thick in the lung periphery. They lie at right angles to the pleura and are best seen near the costophrenic angles. These are caused by fluid in the septa and are called septal lines (formerly known as Kerley B lines). The fluid also causes loss of

---

3 From the Latin *reticulum* = small net.

clarity of the vessel walls. These are the appearances of an interstitial lung disease, acute and diffuse. As the hydrostatic pressure increases the fluid spills over into the pleural spaces and fissures, resulting in pleural effusions.

Congestive cardiac failure (of the left ventricle) of greater severity causes fluid to enter the alveoli from the interstitial space. This appears as consolidation in an X-ray, typically in a perihilar distribution.

2. Chronic interstitial disease

*Localized* disease occurs with entities such as bronchiectasis. The small abscesses that form around the cystic and saccular dilated bronchi heal with scarring of the interstitium. Scarring from previous inflammation is often linear and is a cause of localized, chronic interstitial disease. Radiation fibrosis is another example.

*Diffuse*, chronic disease is what many clinicians are referring to when they speak of 'interstitial lung disease'. There are over 100 causes (groan!) but only five major types (hurrah!). The diseases cause thickening of the lung interstitium with fluid, cellular infiltrate, and connective tissue proliferation. The appearances are those of lines, nodules (<5 mm in diameter), and, in the end stages, a honeycomb appearance of thick walls surrounding grape-like clusters of spaces up to 1 cm in diameter. This honeycomb pattern is actual fibrosis— which is collagenous tissue behaving as a scar does anywhere in the body, contracting as it forms, decreasing the lung volume.

The five main types are:

(a) environmental disease such as coal workers' pneumoconiosis, silicosis, and asbestosis (24%), now fortunately becoming less common;

(b) sarcoidosis (20%), a granulomatous disease of unknown aetiology;

(c) idiopathic pulmonary fibrosis, also called usual interstitial pneumonitis (UIP), or cryptogenic (footnote 4) fibrosing alveolitis (15%). Cryptogenic and idiopathic mean of unknown aetiology. However, the aetiology of the confusing names is known—it reflects different approaches from both sides of the Atlantic and the difficulty in categorizing the disease;

(d) collagen vascular disorders (8%), autoimmune disorders, such as rheumatoid arthritis, and systemic lupus erythematosis;

(e) chronic left heart failure.

The other causes are individually much rarer.

Straight lines are also caused by linear or plate atelectasis and by fibrosis/ scarring.

Lines in the lung may also be curvilinear and circular.

Examples of curvilinear lines are the thick lines of the wall of an abscess or of a cavitating neoplasm. Thin curvilinear lines form the walls of cavities such as the bullae of emphysema or lung cysts.

---

4 From the Greek *kryptos* = hidden.

Question: How can Superman have X-ray vision if X-rays are a transmission image, not reflective?

Bronchial walls seen end-on are circular and difficult to see in healthy people. When they are clearly visible it is because of thickening of the wall due to bronchitis or asthma or from the peribronchial thickening of interstitial disease. The most common of these causes is nicotine addiction and its delivery system.

## Radiolucencies

To explain black areas in the lung and hemithorax think of causes from the hilum and out to the chest wall.

- A pulmonary embolus could cause lung oligaemia (footnote 5) (decreased blood volume).
- Destruction of the alveolar walls and formation of bullae with emphysema is the most common cause of radiolucent lungs.
- Air in the pleural cavity.
- Absent breast tissue gives a more diffuse radiolucency.

## Distortion or displacement of a normal structure

If any structure is the wrong shape or in the wrong place there must be a reason and the cause can usually be determined from the film. The first determination is whether the structure is being pushed or pulled from its usual position: pushed by a pneumothorax, pleural effusion, neoplasm, pectus excavatum moving the heart to the left; pulled by lung collapse or scarring. Compare with old films.

## A normal or abnormal CXR—what does it mean?

In some ways, it is more difficult to call a film normal than to diagnose an abnormality.

If the CXR appears normal, it means that:

- there is no pathology;
- the pathology has cleared;
- the pathology is in the very early stages;
- the abnormality has been missed;
- the abnormality is not detectable with a chest X-ray.

This last group includes small pleural effusions, some signs of pulmonary embolism/infarction, small nodules, and sometimes an anterior pneumothorax in a supine patient. In other words the sensitivity of chest X-rays is not 100%. Sensitivity is the percentage of people with the disease who show a positive test.

Sometimes, when the film is abnormal, it may only be possible to make a generic diagnosis such as consolidation. On another occasion, signs of cardiac enlargement and bilateral perihilar consolidation would allow a specific diagnosis of left heart failure. This diagnosis would also be more likely if the X-ray appearances agreed with the clinical findings. In some ways the radiologist has an advantage over a clinician in that he or she can assess a film and then

### Hint

Remember, for example, the most common chest X-ray appearance of pulmonary embolus is a normal film. It is not the most characteristic finding but it is the most common.

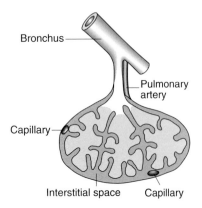

**Fig. 1.14** The acinus and air-space disease. Fluid fills the air spaces.

---

5  From the Greek *oligos* = few, little, less than normal.

subsequently modify that judgement after reading the clinical notes; the film is initially interpreted only on its merits. Clinicians need to be careful not to let their clinical assessment distort the interpretation of what the film displays.

## Summary

When reading a chest X-ray check the identification on the film then study the six areas of interest to find an abnormality. This may take 5 minutes at first but with practice it can be done in 15 seconds. Don't forget that much is learned from a normal film. Every normal radiograph adds information to your mental databank as to what is a usual appearance of someone of that age and sex.

Fluid in the air spaces gives consolidation:
    What are the three types of fluid?
    What are the characteristics of consolidation on a CXR?

Interstitial disease has fluid, ± inflammatory cells, and gives linear ± nodular opacities.

Complete or partial obstruction of a bronchus or bronchiole is caused by something in the lumen, something in the wall, or something outside the wall:
    What are the 5 different appearances complete or partial obstruction can give?

An abnormality will usually allow you to make a generic diagnosis, put you in the ballpark. Comparison with old films, clinical information, and further studies may be needed to make the specific diagnosis. The big question remains, 'Is there enough information to alter the management of the patient or the outcome of the disease?' Read on.

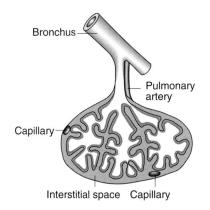

**Fig. 1.15** The acinus and interstitial disease.

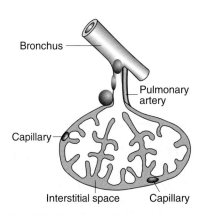

**Fig. 1.16** The acinus and 3 types of obstruction of a bronchus.

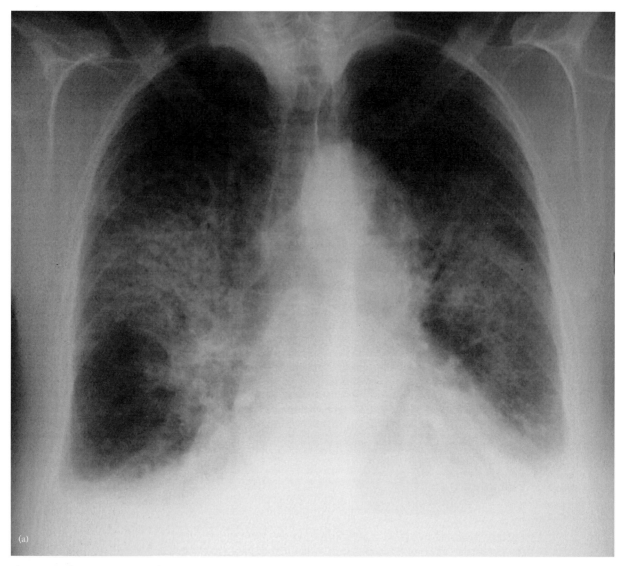

(a)

**Figs 1.17** (a), (b)  Two radiographs, 4 days apart. *Lungs*: The major abnormality in the initial film is in the lungs; perihilar opacities that are poorly defined. This is consolidation. But what is the cause, pulmonary oedema, infection, or blood? The lungs are filled with fluid and unable to expand fully. *Pleura*: The hemidiaphragms are not visible because of pleural effusions, seen curving up the side walls. *Mediastinum*: The heart is enlarged. *Hila, bones, soft tissues*: normal. These are the changes of severe left heart failure. The pulmonary venous pressure has been so high that fluid has flowed from the capillaries, into the interstitium, and then into the alveoli. Look at how the lungs have expanded and the heart borders and hemidiaphragms have sharpened up after treatment.

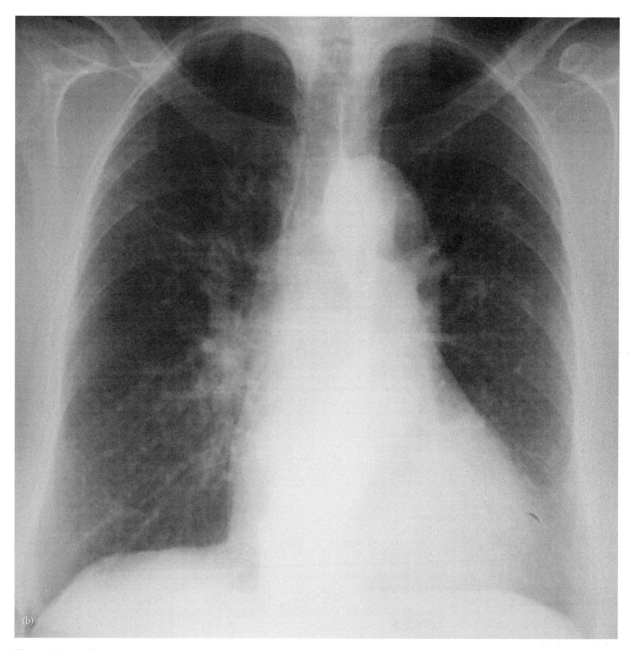

(b)

**Figs** 1.17 *Continued*

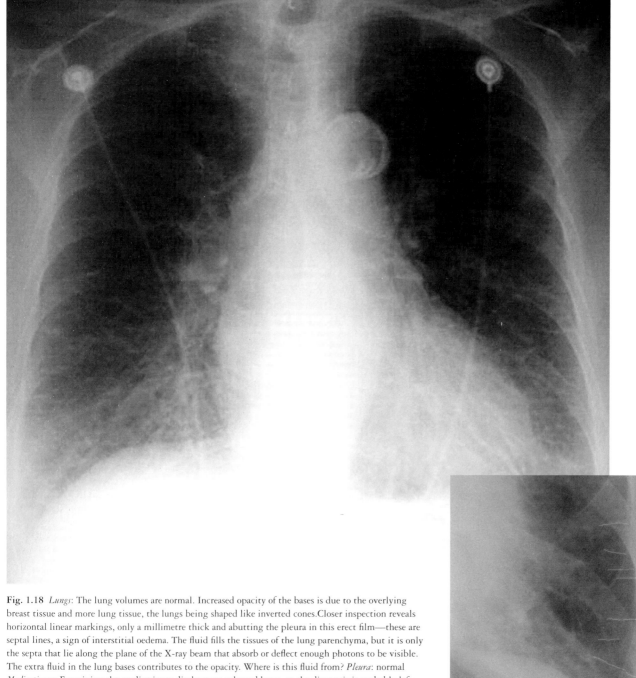

**Fig. 1.18** *Lungs*: The lung volumes are normal. Increased opacity of the bases is due to the overlying breast tissue and more lung tissue, the lungs being shaped like inverted cones.Closer inspection reveals horizontal linear markings, only a millimetre thick and abutting the pleura in this erect film—these are septal lines, a sign of interstitial oedema. The fluid fills the tissues of the lung parenchyma, but it is only the septa that lie along the plane of the X-ray beam that absorb or deflect enough photons to be visible. The extra fluid in the lung bases contributes to the opacity. Where is this fluid from? *Pleura*: normal *Mediastinum*: Examining the mediastinum discloses an enlarged heart, so the diagnosis is probably left heart failure. This is pulmonary venous hypertension, to a moderate degree, displaying interstitial oedema. The increased end-diastolic pressure in the left ventricle has caused increased hydrostatic pressure in the veins and forced fluid from the capillaries into the interstitium. The calcification in the aortic arch gives a clue to the aetiology of the heart failure: atherosclerosis of the coronary arteries. The ECG lines indicate what the clinicians think is the problem. *Hila, bones, soft tissues*: normal.

**Fig. 1.19** Septal lines.

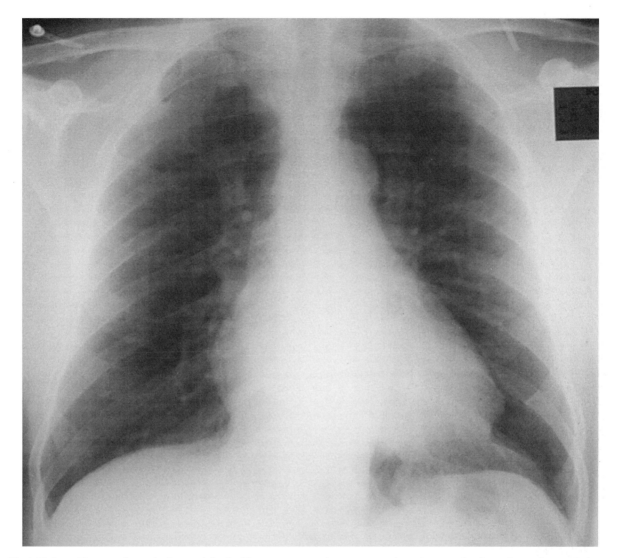

**Fig. 1.20** *Lungs*: These are of normal volume and density. The upper zone vessels are more prominent than normal and are at least as large as the lower zone vessels. It is because the *veins* are big. Normally the upper lobe veins are virtually empty in the erect position but become distended as a result of pulmonary venous hypertension from left heart failure, mitral valve disease, or with lying supine. (Note that pulmonary *arterial* hypertension is a different problem altogether.) This is called upper zone vascular redistribution and is the earliest sign of *left* heart failure. A rule of thumb is that it is present if the veins at the level of the first anterior intercostal space are greater than 3 mm in diameter. The principle of the upper zone veins being distended with left heart failure is similar to that of the jugular venous pressure (JVP) measuring *right* heart failure. *Pleura*: This is normal. *Mediastinum*: heart enlarged. *Hila, bones, soft tissues*: normal. This image and the previous two have demonstrated degrees of cardiac failure. Radionuclear scans, ultrasound, and coronary angiography can assist with estimates of cardiac function and myocardial perfusion.

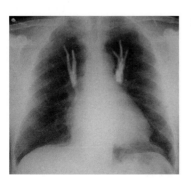

**Fig. 1.21** Upper zone vascular redistribution.

### Hint

Look at a supine film to see *normal* upper zone vascular redistribution.

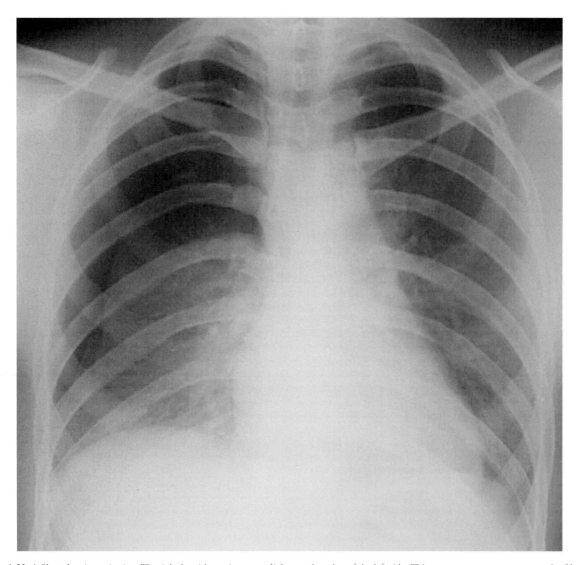

**Fig. 1.22** A film taken in expiration. The right hemithorax is more radiolucent than that of the left side. This appearance can occur as a result of lack of perfusion of the *lung*, destruction of lung tissue, a pneumothorax, loss of soft tissue of the chest wall, or abnormal density of the *left* hemithorax. *Pleura*: The pleural margin of the partly collapsed lung is visible. *Mediastinum*: These structures are unremarkable. *Hila*: The right hilum is depressed. *Bones*: The only bone abnormality is a dysplastic left first rib. *Soft tissues*: normal.

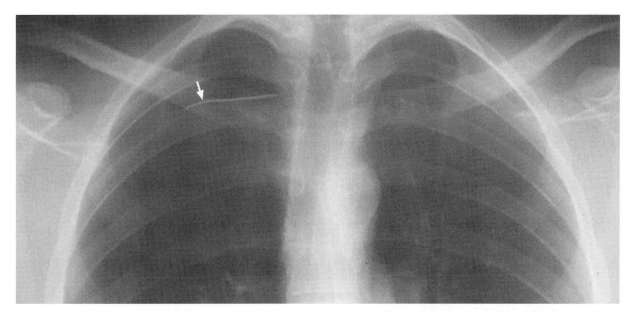

**Fig. 1.23** Less easily seen is the pleural edge superimposed on a rib. No lung markings are visible superior to the right 4th rib. A smaller pneumothorax than in the previous film. The medial border of the right scapula should not be confused with a pleural margin.

*Hint*

Count the ribs starting with the first rib anteriorly, follow it around to the back, and then the second, third, and fourth become distinct.

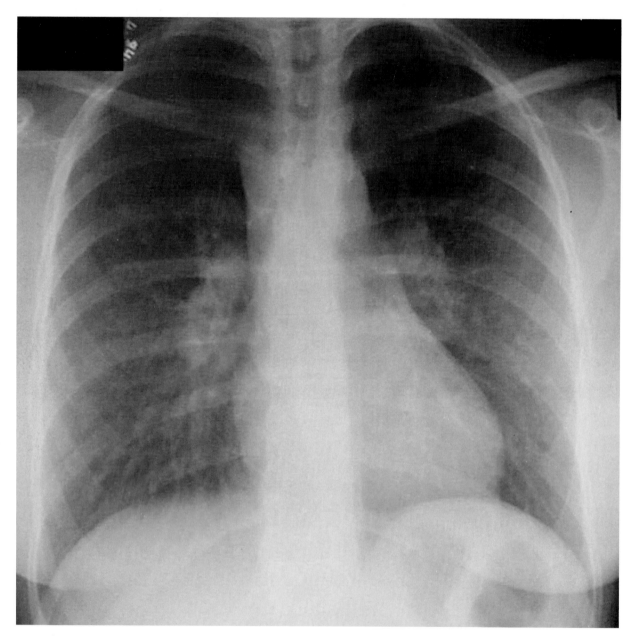

**Fig. 1.24** *Lungs*: normal volume and density. *Pleura*: normal. *Mediastinum*: The paratracheal tissues are prominent. The trachea, left and right main bronchi, aortic arch, and heart are normal. *Hila*: Both are enlarged with nodular, soft-tissue masses. Detecting enlarged hila is a real skill that, like seeing bronchial wall thickening, comes only with practice. *Bones, soft tissues*: normal. Sarcoidosis causes bilateral hila enlargement and mediastinal masses like this. Other diseases to consider in the differential diagnosis are lymphoma and infections, such as infectious mononucleosis. When TB causes lymph-node enlargement, it is unilateral.

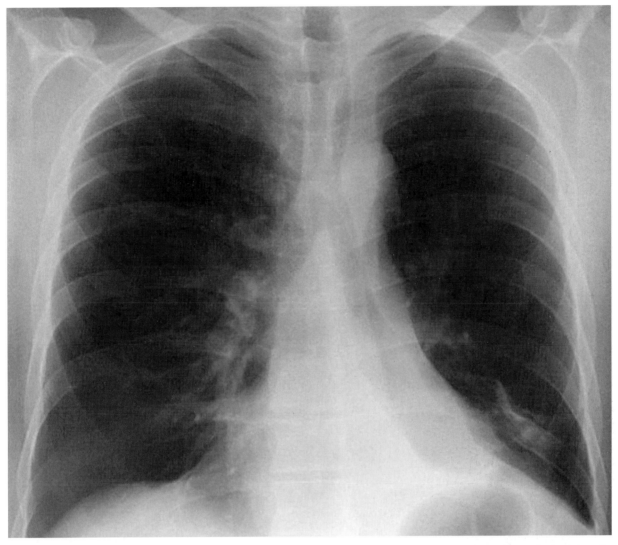

**Fig. 1.25** *Lungs*: These are of normal volume. Fewer markings are seen in the left lung except at the base. *Pleura*: Following the pleura reveals loss of the clarity of the left hemidiaphragm. *Mediastinum*: In the mediastinum the left main bronchus is pulled down and there is a triangular opacity behind the heart on the left. This is a collapsed left lower lobe. It also depresses the left *hilum*. *Bones*: Check the bones for metastatic disease because the left lower lobe bronchus may be obstructed by a neoplasm. *Soft tissues*: appear unremarkable.

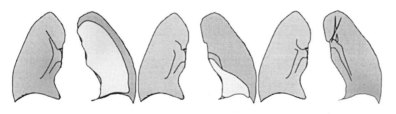

**Fig. 1.26** Types and causes of atelectasis synonym: collapse.

| Pneumothorax and relaxation atelectasis | Obstruction of the bronchus and collapse of the left lower lobe | Fibrosis/scarring of the lung at the left apex. Elevation of the left hilum. Previous TB |

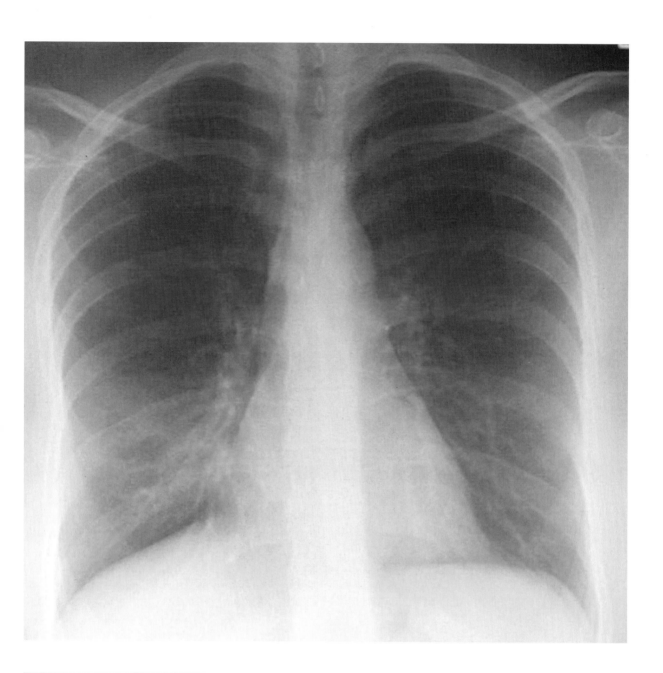

## Hint

With asthma always look carefully at the trachea. Detecting an endobronchial adenoma which can mimic asthma can be life-saving.

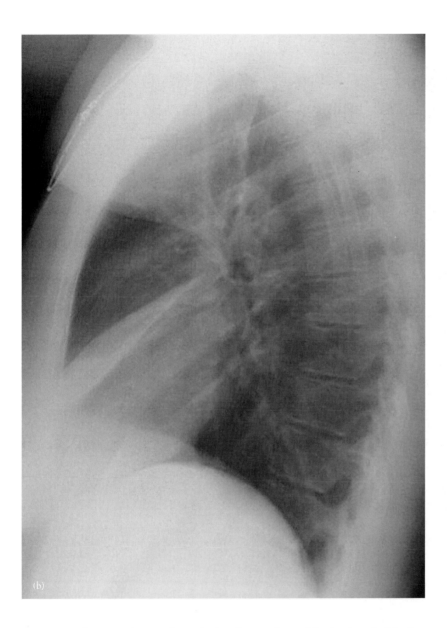

**Figs 1.27** (a), (b) *Lungs*: These are of normal volume but not of normal density. A poorly defined opacity is present at the right base. *Pleura*: Following the pleura around indicates two changes: a positive silhouette sign with loss of the right heart border and elevation of the medial end of the right hemidiaphragm. *Mediastinum*: The heart is part of the mediastinum and is shifted to the right side. *Hila*: The hila are normal, but near the right hilum is a bronchus seen end-on. It has a thickened wall, indicating asthma or bronchitis. *Bones, soft tissues*: normal. The lateral CXR shows the pathology more clearly because the collapsed middle lobe is seen in profile. The horizontal and oblique fissures are approximated. The aetiology of the collapse must be something in the bronchial lumen, in the wall, or something outside the wall. The history would give the clue, but the radiologist could use two pieces of information to arrive at the correct answer: (a) thickened bronchial walls; (b) the epidemiology. The most common cause of a collapsed lobe in a woman of this age, 30, is asthma, secondary to mucous plugging.

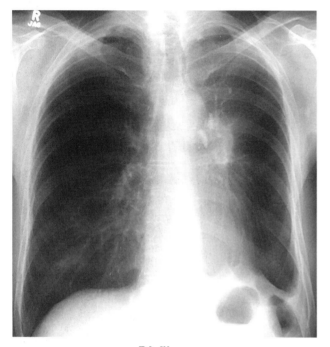

**PA film**

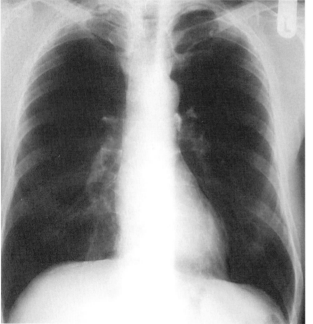

**Three years ago**

[Lateral film image]

**Lateral film**

**Fig. 1.28** *Lungs*: The left hemithorax has an increased density and decreased volume. *Pleura*: Searching the outlines of the pleura uncovers elevation of the left hemidiaphragm, a left pleural effusion, and loss of the clarity of the aortic arch, main pulmonary artery, and the left heart border. *Mediastinum*: The trachea and the heart are shifted to the left. Is the mediastinum being pushed to the left by some right-sided pathology or pulled by pathology in the left lung? The loss of clarity of the aortic arch and left heart border together with a loss of volume indicates a left upper lobe collapse, and this is confirmed on the lateral view. The lobe has collapsed forward and superiorly. Two calcified nodes are also present, a result of previous TB infection. *Hila*: The soft tissue mass in the left *hilum* was shown to be a carcinoma. *Bones, soft tissues*: normal. Fibrotic changes have caused tenting, 'tethering' of the left hemidiaphragm. When an abnormality is found, compare with a previous film.

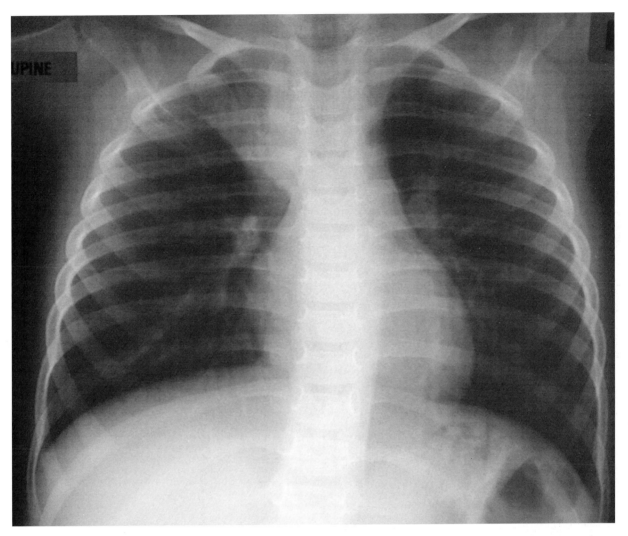

**Fig. 1.29** Several factors in the young child's anatomy contribute to a different appearance of the chest X-ray:

- relatively larger heart and vessels;
- higher diaphragm position (larger abdominal organs; children under the age of 5 years are often X-rayed lying supine);
- broader and shorter chest shape;
- large thymus which is often very prominent up to 1 year of age but may be visible up to 6 years.

The *lungs* are at least at the upper limit of normal size for a 3-year-old child. The problem is to work out what is the opacity in the right apex. The horizontal fissure has been pulled up. The clarity of the *pleural* edge of the right paratracheal line is lost and the pathology appears contiguous with the superior *mediastinum*. *Hila, bones, soft tissues*: normal. The opacity in the right upper zone is the right upper lobe, collapsed against the mediastinum. In this child the cause is likely to be mucous plugging from asthma.

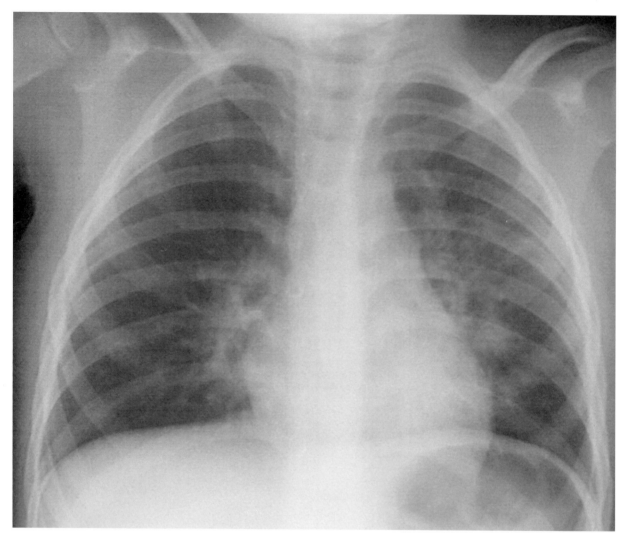

**Fig.** 1.30 *Lungs*: They are of normal volume in this 4-year-old child, but demonstrate poorly defined opacities in the perihilar regions. *Pleura*: The pleural edge along the left heart border is not clearly demonstrated. *Mediastinum*: The mediastinal abnormality is a density behind the heart. *Hila*: These are obscured by the increased density that, on closer observation, consists of thickened bronchial walls. *Bones, soft tissues*: normal. This appearance is called perihilar inflammatory changes and is a result of infection/bronchitis and perhaps a degree of asthma. The changes can persist, becoming chronic. For this reason a follow-up film is not always helpful.

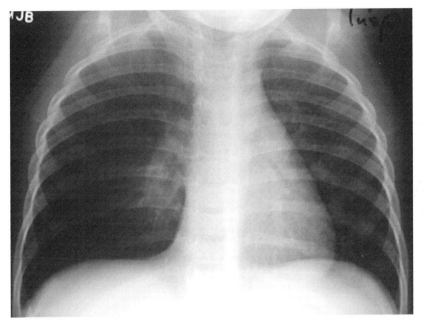

**Inspiration**

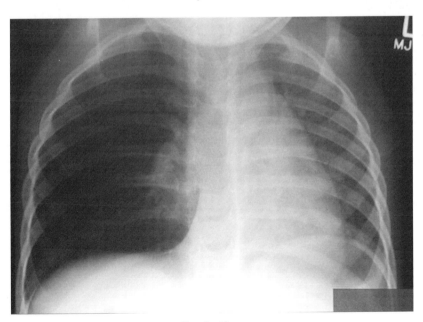

**Expiration**

**Fig.** 1.31 (a) In the inspiratory film the right *lung* is larger than the left. The *pleura* is normal. The right lung appears hyperexpanded because the *mediastinum* is shifted to the left and the hemidiaphragm is depressed. No significant abnormality of the *hila, bones,* or *soft tissues*. (b) With expiration, the left lung becomes smaller but the right lung remains the same size. It seems that the right main bronchus is obstructed, air getting in but not getting out. Inhalation of a peanut has caused this. Air can get past the obstruction on inspiration. With expiration, the diameter of the bronchus decreases, trapping the air, a condition known as obstructive emphysema.

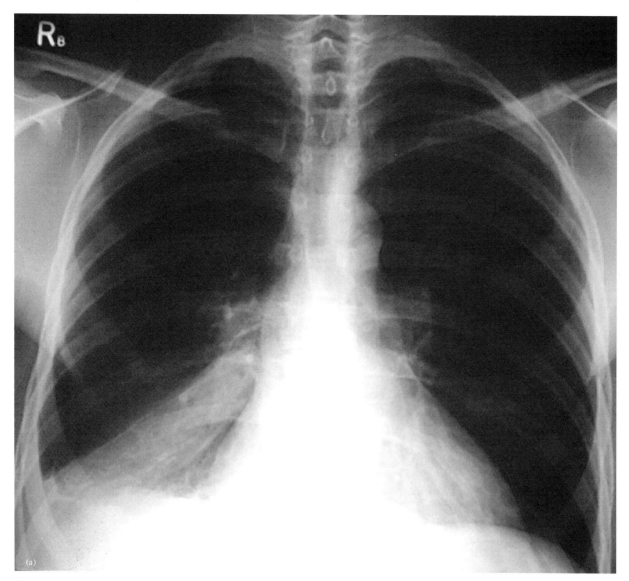

(a)

**Figs 1.32** (a), (b) *Lungs*: The abnormality is at the base of the right lung. Closer observation of this large opacity should reveal if it is consolidation, collapse, or pleural fluid. The straight edge of the opacity is the oblique fissure that has been rotated and pulled down by loss of volume of the right lower lobe. *Pleura*: The pleural outline at the right costophrenic angle and over the hemidiaphragm is lost because of a pleural effusion, seen extending up the chest wall. *Mediastinum*: The abnormality is increased density behind the right side of the heart. *Hila, bones, soft tissues*: Look at these particularly for signs of metastatic disease. In the lateral X-ray the vertebral bodies are relatively opaque in the lower chest. Only one hemidiaphragm, the left, is visible. This is an example of collapse of the right lower lobe and a pleural effusion. There should be no effusion with asthma. Bronchoscopy is indicated to find the cause.

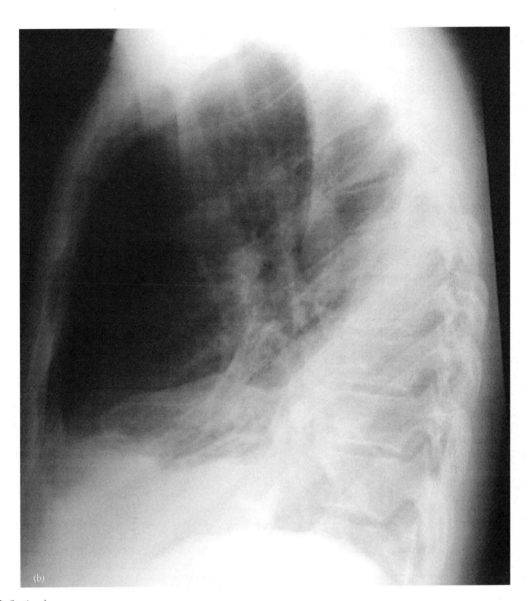

(b)

**Figs 1.32** *Continued*

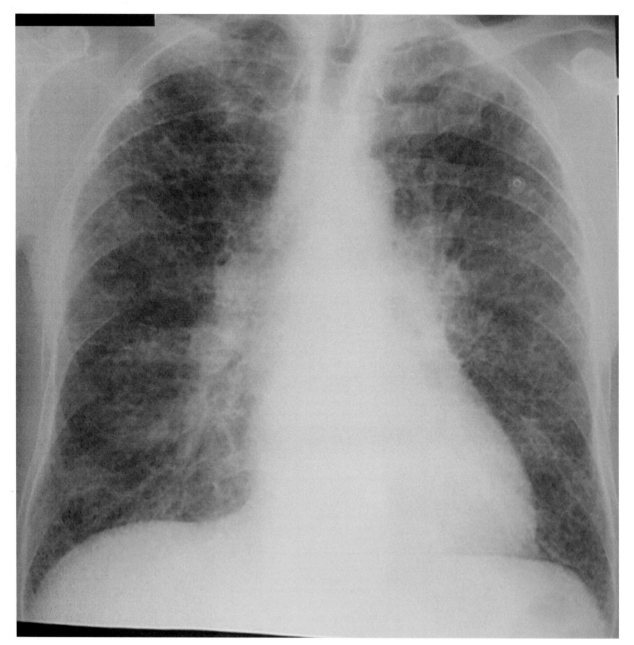

**Fig. 1.33** *Lungs*: The lungs are of normal volume but have a generalized increase in markings. These are both linear and reticular and you are thinking 'are they acute or chronic?' *Pleura*: The pleural lining lacks clarity as a result of the lung disease. *Mediastinum*: normal. *Hila*: These are prominent as a result of large pulmonary arteries, reflecting pulmonary arterial hypertension caused by the lung changes. *Bones, soft tissues*: normal. If this were acute, it would probably be left heart failure. But you called for the old films and realized it was unchanged over the last 3 years. It is therefore a chronic interstitial lung disease and should be one of the five common types. An open biopsy diagnosed asbestosis, one of the pneumoconioses. These fibrotic lung diseases can cause small lung volumes or, as in this case, destroy the elastic tissue and have normal lung volumes. The actual disease of *asbestosis* is one of fibrosis of the lungs, usually at the bases. Pleural plaques, whether calcified or not, can occur as a result of a haemothorax, empyema, or after *exposure* to asbestos.

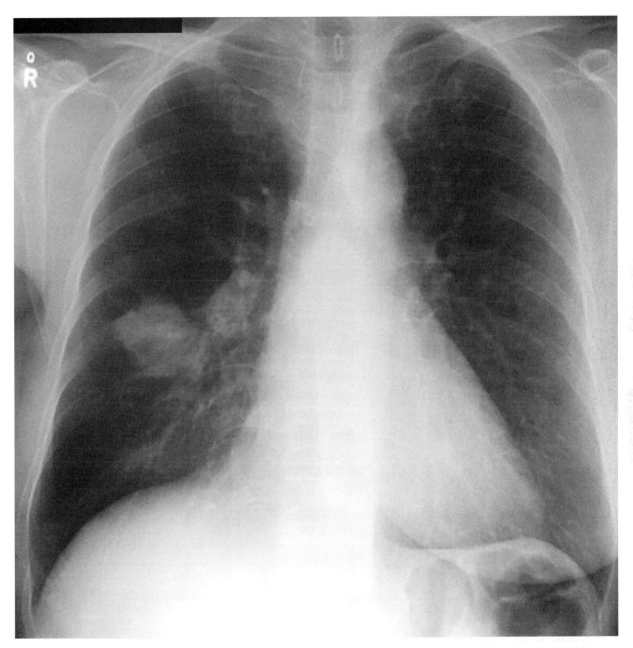

**Fig. 1.34** *Lungs*: The lungs demonstrate two abnormalities. The right lung appears more radiolucent than the left and there is a well-defined, but irregularly shaped, mass in the right mid-zone. *Pleura*: normal *Mediastinum*: normal structures *Hila*: The right *hilum* is made prominent by a mass. *Bones*: normal *Soft tissues*: Examination reveals the cause of the radiolucency of the right lung to be a mastectomy. Your thinking will go like this: A mass in the right lung and another in the hilum. Probably secondary carcinoma from the breast. Comparison with previous films would be useful in the first instance. Further investigation with CT of the chest, bronchoscopy, and fine-needle aspiration may be warranted.

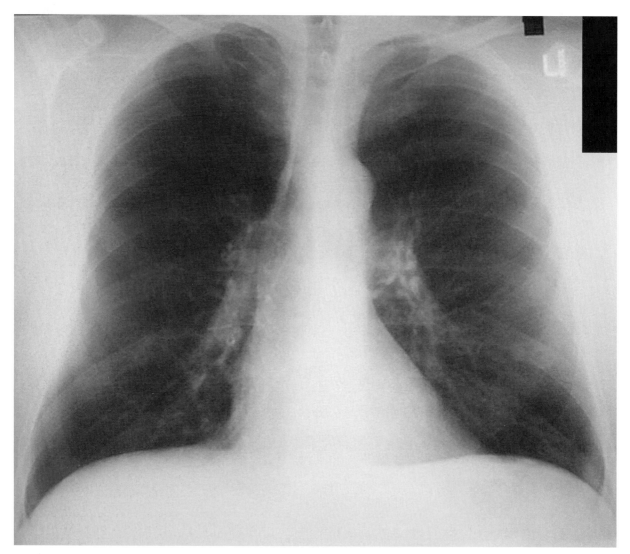

**Fig. 1.35** This X-ray is typical of what is seen when a person presents with a history of chronic cough or vague chest pain. It is often not of much help except to exclude cardiac failure, infection, or neoplasm. *Lungs*: The lungs show increased markings. When that occurs look for thickening of the bronchial walls as that is the most common cause and can be a result of cigarette smoking, inflammation from infection or asthma, or early pulmonary oedema. Two bronchi with thickened walls are seen end-on near the right hilum. *Pleura*: normal *Mediastinum*: normal structures *Hila*: The hila are prominent because of large pulmonary arteries. Why are they large? Because of inflammation and destruction of the lung tissue, causing increased peripheral resistance and pulmonary *arterial* hypertension. *Bones*, *soft tissues*: normal. The diagnosis is chronic lung disease, probably a mixture of bronchitis and emphysema.

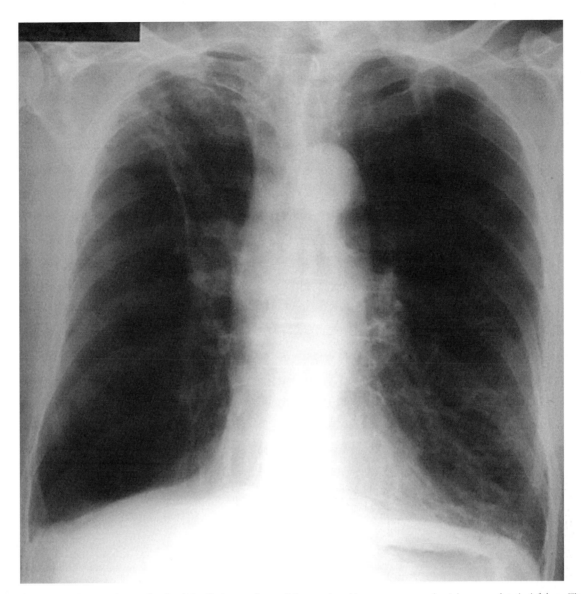

**Fig. 1.36** *Lungs*: The lungs are hyperinflated and the diaphragms flattened. Increased markings are present at the right apex and at the left base. The remainder of the lungs appears radiolucent. Why is this so? Let us first check the other areas. *Pleura*: Pleural thickening is seen at the right apex. *Mediastinum*: This is normal for a person of this age (75 years), or even a little narrow because of the depressed diaphragm. *Hila*: The right hilum has been pulled up by the changes at the apex, fibrosis caused by tuberculosis (footnote 6). *Bones, soft tissues*: Seem to be normal. The changes at the left base look like crowding of the vessels. This is a type of relaxation atelectasis caused by destruction of lung parenchyma in the upper zone. The destruction is likely to be of the alveolar walls distal to the terminal bronchioles, that is, emphysema. The remaining elastic tissue in the lower zone results in approximation of the vessels and airways. Comparison with old films would be useful. Any suggestion of recent change in the scarring at the right apex would require sputum cultures to exclude active TB.

---

6 *Primary TB* shows as consolidation in the lung mid-zone, called a Ghon focus, and an accompanying unilateral lymph node enlargement in the hilum. If both are present it is called a Ghon complex. Somehow and sometimes the acid-fast bacilli reach the upper lobes and *postprimary TB* then occurs at a later date. Consolidation develops and heals with scarring and calcification in the lung apices. Radiological signs of TB therefore are consolidation, lymph node enlargement, pleural effusion, apical lung fibrosis, cavity formation, and calcification. Distant spread occurs if the body's defences are overcome: the bone destruction of osteomyelitis which can be devastating in the thoracolumbar spine; scarring of the kidney and ureter; involvement of the meninges; or a shower of blood-borne organisms seen as miliary TB in the lungs.

When scarring is seen in the upper zones of the lungs it is usually due to TB or radiotherapy.

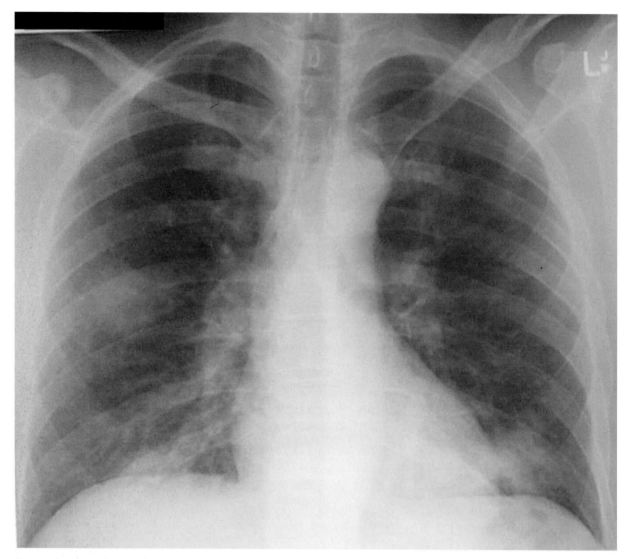

**Fig. 1.37** *Lungs*: The lungs are of normal volume, but five poorly defined opacities are visible. *Pleura*: The pleural margin is blurred (positive silhouette sign) at the left heart border and over part of the right hemidiaphragm indicating, without need of a lateral film, that the pathology is in the lungs. *Mediastinum, hila*: normal *Bones* and *soft tissues*: These are also unremarkable except for an old fracture of the left clavicle. The opacities are poorly defined and with no loss of volume, indicating consolidation, even though there is no evidence of air-bronchograms or limitation by the fissures. This is bronchopneumonia. It might be regarded as a development of bronchitis, caused by a more aggressive organism or with less host resistance.

## In the following films look for these features:

- poorly defined opacity;
- limited by a fissure;
- air bronchogram;
- no loss of volume.

If some of these are present it means consolidation and could be due to pneumonia, oedema, or blood in the alveoli.

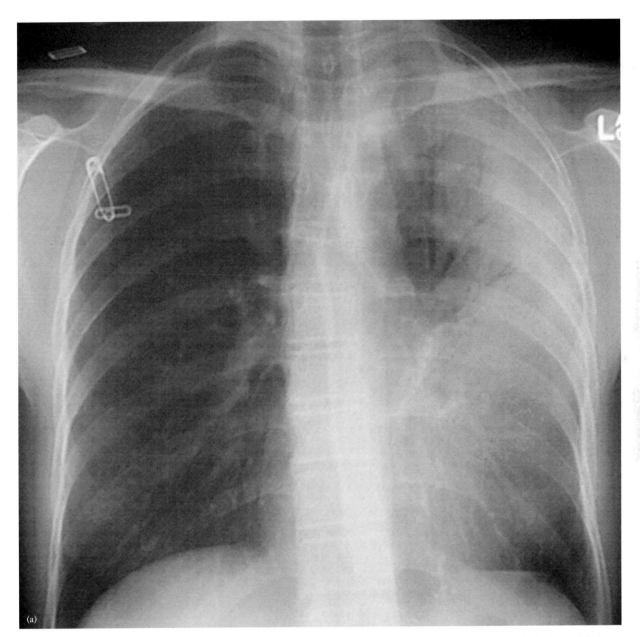

(a)

**Figs 1.38** (a), (b)

*Lungs*: Normal lung volumes. A poorly defined opacity in the left lung obliterates the left heart border and therefore is in the upper lobe. The air-bronchogram indicates consolidation. *Pleura*: The pleura in the right hemithorax seems normal. *Mediastinum*: This is central but the oblique fissure on the lateral film is bowed inferiorly because of a slight increase in volume. *Hila*: The left hilum is not visible. *Bones, soft tissues*: normal. Left upper lobe pneumonia (lobar pneumonia). Pneumonia is an infection of the lung, classified as lobar, broncho, and atypical. Usually the pathology progresses through four stages: congestion, red hepatization, grey hepatization, and resolution. This would be one of the stages of hepatization.

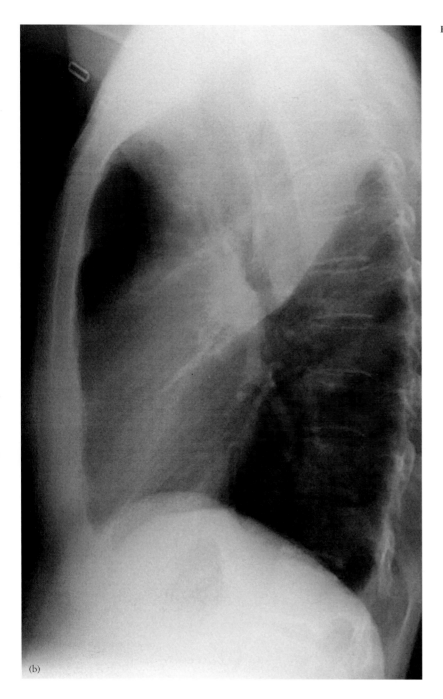

(b)

Figs 1.38 (continued)

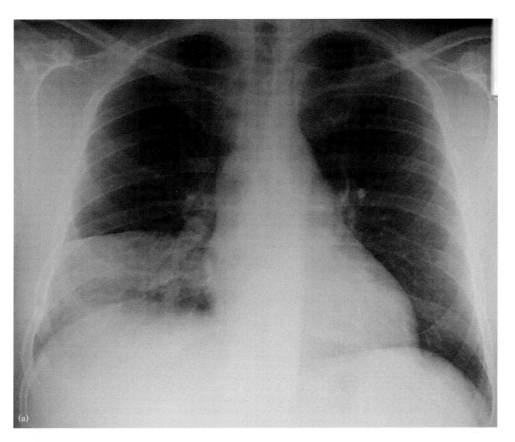

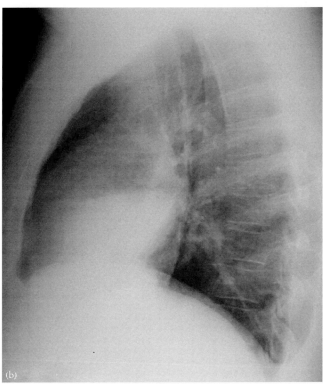

**Figs 1.39** (a), (b) *Lungs*: An opacity can be seen at the base of the right lung. *Pleura*: The silhouette of the pleura over the right hemidiaphragm is lost because of adjacent lung disease. The right heart border is also unclear. *Mediastinum, hila, bones, soft tissues*: normal. The middle lobe has two segments. The consolidation of lobar pneumonia here involves principally the lateral segment. The medial segment is affected to a lesser extent, shown by the loss of clarity of the right heart border. Also well seen on the lateral projection, but the PA view has adequate information.

**Figs** 1.40 (a), (b) Original films; (c), (d) 2 weeks later. *Lungs*: A poorly defined opacity can be seen at the left lung base. *Pleura*: Looking at the pleura discloses elevation of the left hemidiaphragm. *Mediastinum, hila, bones, soft tissues*: all normal. On the lateral film the *retrosternal space* is normal, as is the *subcarinal region*. The *vertebral bodies* do not become more black as the diaphragm is approached. One of the hemidiaphragms is obscured posteriorly so that one *costophrenic angle* is not visible. The left hemidiaphragm is the one that is not seen. It is the one usually not visible as far forward as that on the right side because the heart obscures the left hemidiaphragm silhouette anteriorly. Left lower lobe pneumonia. But consider pulmonary infarction and haemorrhage as a cause. Compare the appearances with the film taken 2 weeks later.

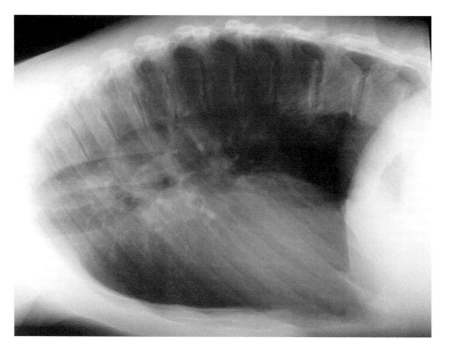

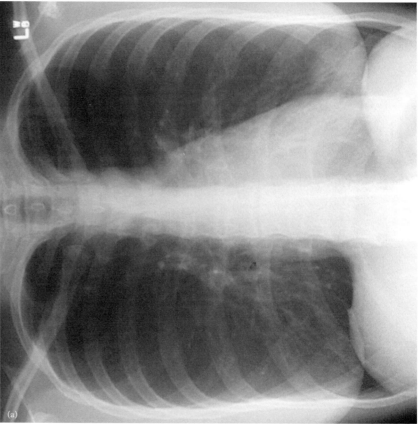

(a)

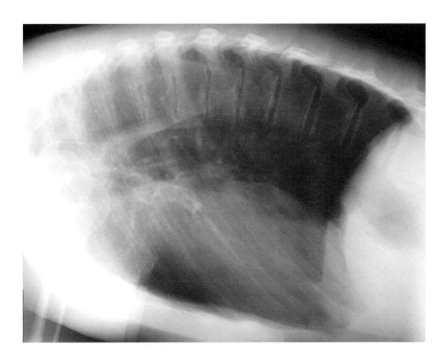

Figs 1.40 *Continued*

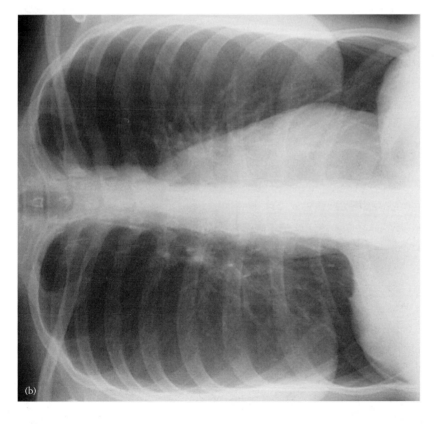

(b)

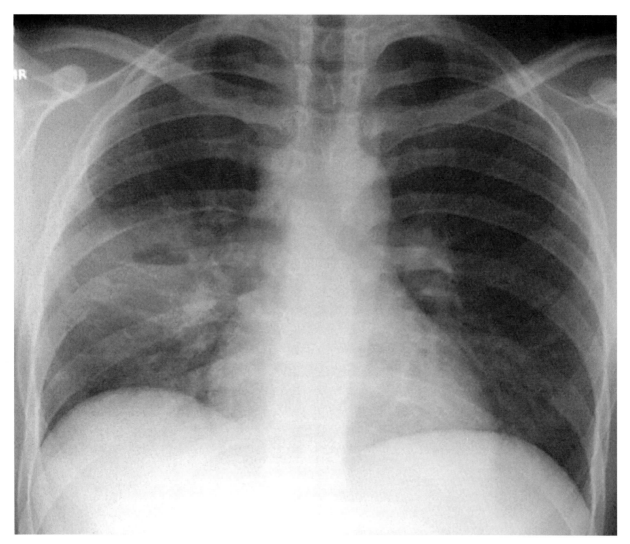

**Fig.** 1.41 A film taken in expiration because of right-sided chest pain, thought to be a pneumothorax. *Lungs*: A poorly defined opacity occupies the mid-zone of the right lung. *Pleura, mediastinum, hila, bones, soft tissues*: None of these add any clues to the diagnosis. The opacity is consolidation and demonstrates a complication. An aggressive infection by bacteria can sometimes attack the blood vessels, causing vasculitis with ischaemia and infarction of the affected tissue, a lung abscess. Some of the necrotic tissue has been discharged into a bronchus and coughed up. In return, air has entered the cavity, which now shows an air-fluid level with this horizontal beam film. Cavities also can develop in a primary or secondary neoplasm, particularly squamous cell carcinoma.

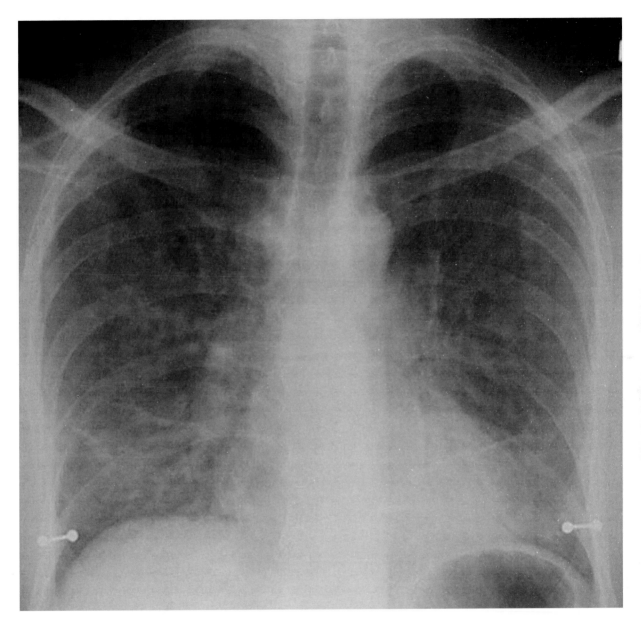

**Fig. 1.42** *Lungs*: They have signs both of consolidation and of an increase of linear markings. *Pleura* and *mediastinum*: The pleural outline over the left hemidiaphragm is lost and when looking at the mediastinum one sees the increased density of the left side of the heart, indicating consolidation at the left base posteriorly. *Hila, bones*: These add no more information. *Soft tissues*: The abnormality is studs in the nipples. This 38-year-old man is immuno-compromised. The appearances are those of an infection (pneumonia) that has spread through the lung without much host resistance. In this case it was caused by *Legionella micdadei*. The body's defences can be severely reduced by AIDS, leukaemia, or chemotherapy and many unusual organisms flourish. TB should be considered in the differential diagnosis.

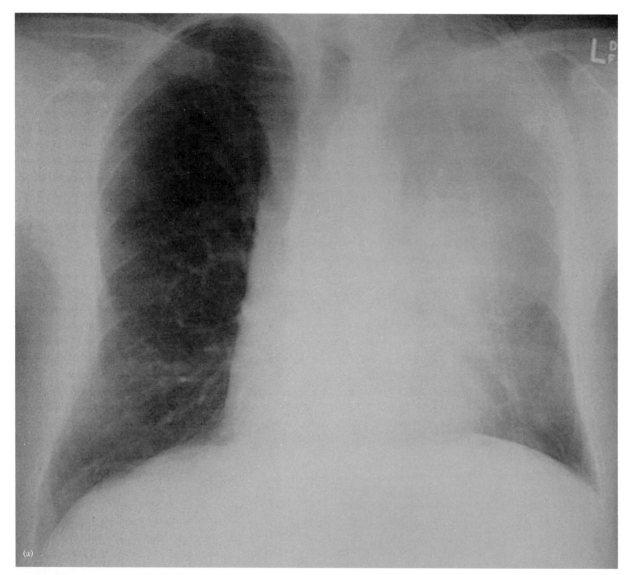

(a)

**Figs** 1.43 (a) (b) It takes one nanosecond to see that this is an abnormal CXR, but longer to work out what is the problem. On the other hand, it can take a minute or two to call a film normal. A large opacity occupies the upper- and mid-zones of the left hemithorax. *Lungs*: The left lung volume is reduced, shown by mild elevation of the hemidiaphragm. *Pleura* and *mediastinum*: Following the pleura discloses loss of the left mediastinal border, particularly of the left heart. The mediastinal structures are not displaced. *Hila*: These are not clearly visible. *Bones*: No sign of destructive lesions. *Soft tissues*: normal. The lateral film confirms the opacity to be in the left upper lobe and is limited by the oblique fissure. It looks like consolidation but there is no air-bronchogram. The diagnosis is obstructive pneumonitis, one of the results of obstruction of a bronchus. Fluid from the lining cells has filled both the airways (air passages) and air spaces (alveoli and alveolar sacs) distal to the obstruction. The diagnosis is carcinoma of the upper lobe bronchus with involvement of the phrenic nerve causing elevation of the hemidiaphragm. There is not yet enough information to take action (start treatment). Seek diagnostic cells with a bronchoscopy and determine the extent of the tumour with a CT of the chest and liver.

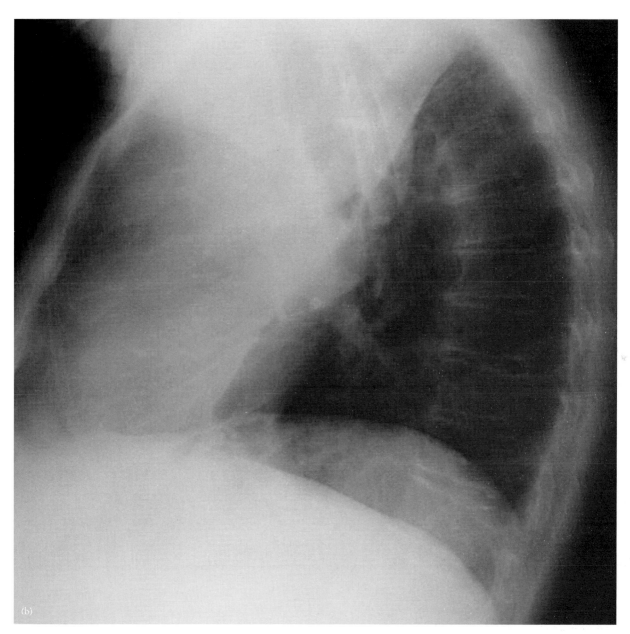

**Figs 1.43** *Continued*

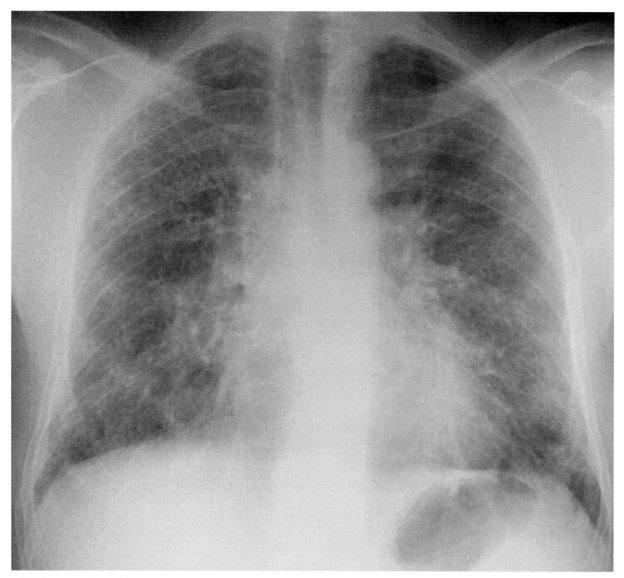

**Fig. 1.44** *Lungs*: The lung volumes are normal but the parenchyma shows increased markings that extend out to the chest wall. Normally vessels (arteries and veins) are only seen for 80% of the distance from hilum to pleura. The bronchi should barely be visible. *Pleura*: Following the pleura demonstrates that the heart borders are poorly defined, reflecting interstitial disease in the lung adjacent to the heart. *Mediastinum*: The mediastinal structures themselves are normal. *Hila*: The hila are difficult to interpret. So what? It is not unusual to be missing a piece of information when making a clinical decision. No need for wringing of hands and gnashing of teeth. Either go ahead without it or, if it is essential, find it. In this case, further information is available by comparison with old films or by requesting a CT. *Bone* and *soft tissues*: No abnormality. This is interstitial lung disease. It has a similar appearance to the interstitial oedema of moderate left heart failure but without a big heart. Check the previous film to see if it is acute. It was not. The diagnosis in this example is fibrosing alveolitis

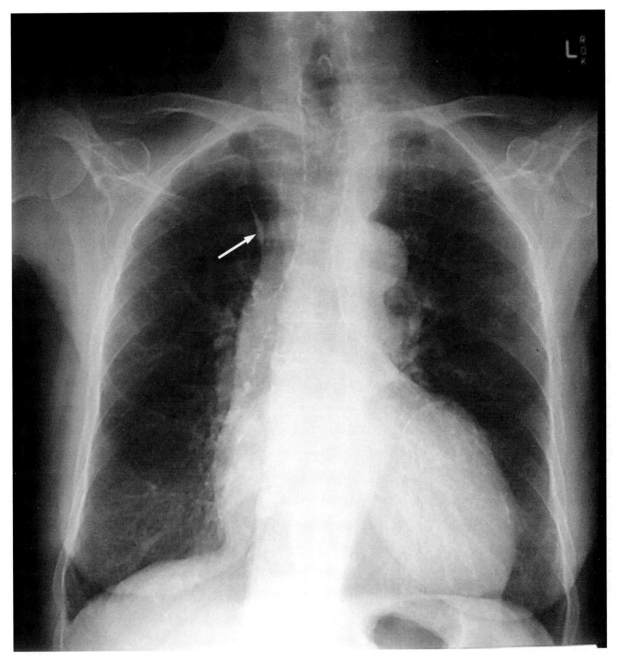

**Fig. 1.45** This is a typical film of an elderly person. *Lungs*: The lungs have gradually expanded over the years because of the loss of elastic tissue, same mechanism as wrinkles developing in the skin. In the right upper zone is a normal variant. It is the azygos vein, seen inferiorly in the azygos fissure (arrow) instead of being at the angle of the trachea and right main bronchus. *Pleura*: The pleura is unremarkable. *Mediastinum*: Some widening of the upper mediastinum is allowed because of the tortuosity of the brachiocephalic and left subclavian arteries. The cardiac silhouette is enlarged but there is no other evidence of cardiac insufficiency (a more gentle term than failure), such as pulmonary oedema. The bulge on the left border of the heart has peripheral calcification and is likely to be a ventricular aneurysm, present for some time. *Hila*: normal *Bones*: Degenerative change in the right acromioclavicular joint is the only bone abnormality. *Soft tissues*: normal. So what's the diagnosis? If there wasn't a ventricular aneurysm you could call this film normal for age.

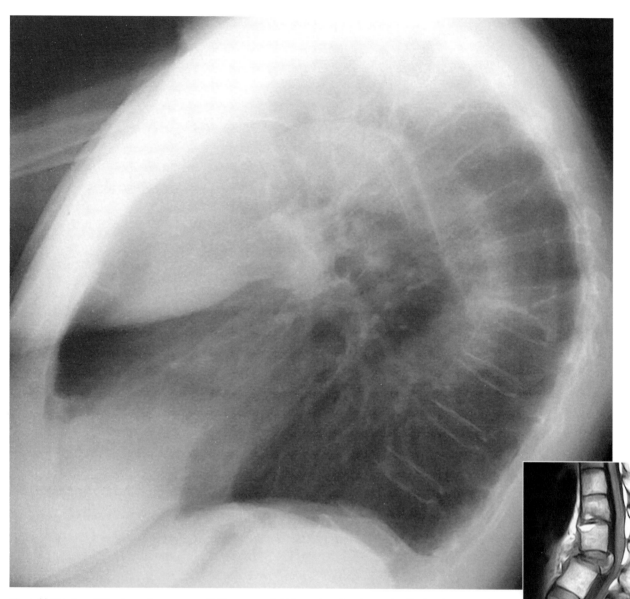

**Fig. 1.46** This lateral film shows the anatomy well. The arms are held forward to allow better visualization, but some of the soft tissue of the arms covers part of the *retrosternal space*. Follow the line of the trachea down to the *subcarinal region*. The *vertebral bodies* should become more radiolucent from above, down to the diaphragm. When one looks for this, a wedge fracture of the T7 vertebral body is apparent. All the vertebrae have the loss of density and thinned cortex typical of osteoporosis. One of the *posterior costophrenic angles* is blunted from a small pleural effusion or pleural thickening. The significant complication of a wedge or compression fracture is narrowing of the spinal canal by a bone fragment protruding posteriorly. MRI or CT examination can confirm or exclude compression of the thecal sac and spinal cord.

**Fig. 1.47** An axial loading injury caused this compression fracture of L1. The retropulsed fragment of the vertebral body compresses the distal spinal cord (grey). The CSF is black and the fat in the bone marrow and subcutaneous tissues is white—a T1-weighted scan. The T11–T12 disc is also damaged.

## CT of the chest

*Some simple rules for looking at the CT chest images*

Where to look:

(1) lungs

## What to look for (lungs)

*Opacity:*

- interstitial disease (reticular or nodular), lung masses, air-space disease

*Radiolucency:*

- destructive changes (emphysema, bullae, cysts)

*Distortion or displacement:*

- dilated bronchi, thickened walls

(2) mediastinum

## What to look for (mediastinum)

*Opacity:*

- neoplastic mass, enlarged node

*Radiolucency:*

- gas

*Distortion or displacement of a structure:*

- displacement of the mediastinum or any of its components, aortic aneurysm, enlarged heart

(3) chest wall

## What to look for (chest wall)

*Opacity:*

- nodes in the axilla

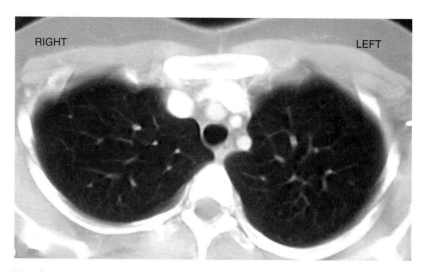

**Fig. 1.48** Consider that you are standing at the foot of the patient. This is a reference slice in CT of the thorax. It is at the level of the manubrium, just below the sternoclavicular joints. The left brachiocephalic vein arches across anteriorly to join the right brachiocephalic vein. Behind the left vein are three arteries—the brachiocephalic, left common carotid, and left subclavian—from medial to lateral.

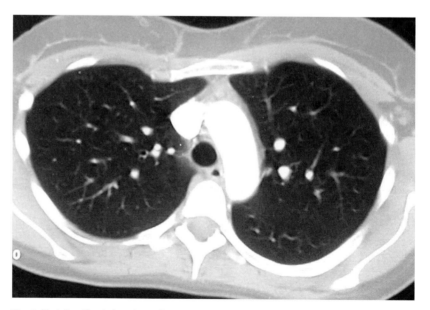

**Fig. 1.49** A few slices inferiorly, the brachiocephalic veins have joined to form the superior vena cava (SVC). The only major vessels seen are the SVC and the aortic arch. The oesophagus, posterior to the trachea, contains some gas.

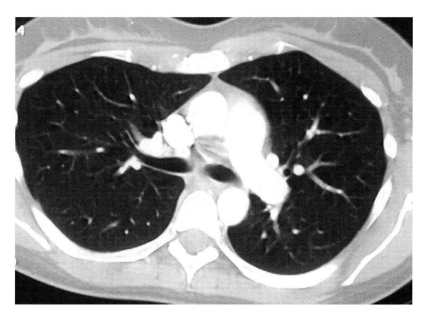

**Fig. 1.50** Follow the SVC. It contains a greater concentration of contrast than the other vessels and causes some artefact. Next to it is the ascending aorta and next to the aorta is the pulmonary artery. The (main) pulmonary artery leads into the left pulmonary artery. The right pulmonary artery lies inferior to this level (remember the CXR appearances). Between the pulmonary artery and the arch of the aorta, superior to this slice, is the space called the aortopulmonary window. We are looking at the inferior boundary of that space. The trachea has divided into the right and left main bronchi. Posterior to the left main bronchus is the descending aorta.

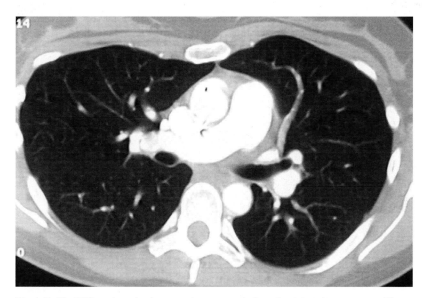

**Fig. 1.51** The SVC continues its descent and passes anteriorly to the right pulmonary artery. The left pulmonary artery has arched over the left main bronchus and the descending branch is visible posterior to the bronchus. Anterior to that bronchus is the superior pulmonary vein, coming down to join the left atrium.

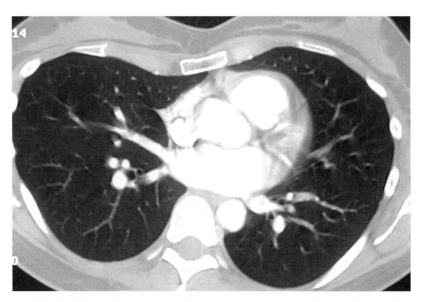

**Fig. 1.52** The SVC is still descending and lies adjacent to the outlet of the left ventricle which, in turn, is next to the right ventricular outlet. Posterior is the left atrium, accepting blood from the inferior pulmonary veins. Part of the wall of this chamber forms the posterior border of the heart on a lateral chest X-ray.

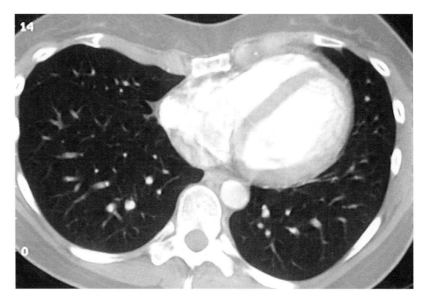

**Fig. 1.53** The SVC has finally joined the right atrium, here contiguous with the right ventricle, the tricuspid valve is not seen. What is visible is the interventricular septum and left ventricle. The left border of the heart is formed by a wall of the left ventricle and the right border by that of the right atrium. As an exercise, follow the path of blood flow down the SVC, then out of the right ventricle, back into the left atrium, and out of the left ventricle.

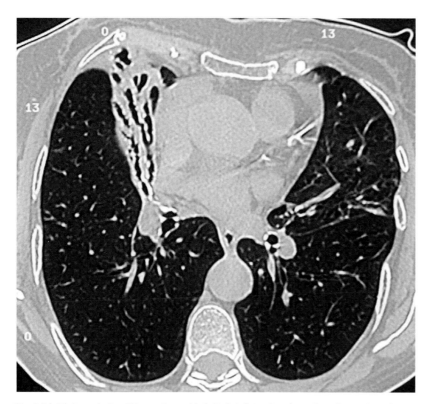

**Fig.** 1.54 High-resolution CT scans have added much information about chest disease since the technology first allowed high-quality scans in the 1980s. This slice is made with an X-ray beam 1 mm thick. The CXR showed an opacity adjacent to the right heart border with loss of the silhouette. The CT allows the diagnosis of bronchiectasis. This disease is irreversible dilatation of the bronchi, caused by, or accompanied, by a chronic, necrotizing infection. The infection in the bronchi has penetrated the walls to form small abscesses which healed with scarring, each episode of acute infection contributing a little. Seen here is the end result of middle lobe involvement, dilated bronchi pulled together by scar tissue. The calcification (white, + artefact) posterior to the pulmonary artery is in the wall of the left coronary artery.

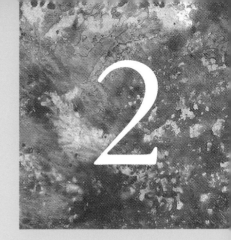

2

# *Abdominal X-rays*

- Systematic approach:
  Gas pattern
  Biliary tree and right urinary tract
  Left urinary tract
  Bones
  Soft tissues
- The common and important abnormalities of the AXR:
  Fluid levels and dilated loops
  Pneumoperitoneum
  Sick bowel
  Calcification

- Summary

# Abdominal X-rays

The main focus of this chapter is to help the reader become competent in interpreting plain abdominal X-rays, learning:

(1) normal radiological anatomy;

(2) how to look at the images:

    (a) where to look:

        (i) following a logical perceptual flow,

        (ii) important sites;

    (b) what to look for:

        (i) abnormal density,

        (ii) abnormal radiolucency,

        (iii) distortion or displacement of a normal structure;

(3) how to interpret the abnormalities by:

    (a) recognizing the abnormality,

    (b) describing it in generic terms,

    (c) giving a specific diagnosis, or

    (d) knowing where to go to acquire that information;

(4) features of several diseases.

This chapter is not a compendium of diseases of the gastrointestinal tract. It cannot give a description of most diseases and how they appear in various modalities. That would require a text of 500 pages.

What it does do is teach the skills to interpret the most common film and the one that may arrive without a radiologist's report.

For other investigations the important knowledge for non-radiologists is when to order radiographs, and the significance of the results. Section 2 provides information about how to order the correct test. It centres on asking the right questions such as, 'What do I need to know?'

## Systematic approach

For abdominal X-rays, devise a system for yourself that covers the documentary evidence of name, age, and technical factors, followed by five areas of interest:

(1) abdominal gas pattern;

(2) biliary tree and right urinary tract;

(3) left urinary tract and bladder;

(4) bones;

(5) soft tissues.

Link each feature to the following one so that a perceptual flow develops. Do not try to cover two areas such as the urinary tract and bones at once.

> ### Hint
> Read this chapter while sitting directly in front of a viewing box or monitor with an abdominal X-ray (AXR) displayed. Optimize the viewing conditions by turning off adjacent lights.

The following section is a description of *one* approach to reading an AXR, having good perceptual flow as well as emphasizing the important structures first.

Each of the five areas is described. Consider when you are looking at these areas that an abnormality can only be one of three things:

- an opacity
- a radiolucency
- distortion or displacement of a normal structure.

Examples of these three groups of abnormalities are presented.

Check the name, age, and whether the film is taken supine or erect. Usually, a supine AXR and an erect CXR are sufficient as the initial investigation. The supine film is easier to read because the abdominal contents are spread out more evenly. Technically, it is a superior film because the abdomen has a relatively uniform thickness when the patient is supine compared to the unevenness caused by gravity as the abdominal wall sags in the erect position. Mammography uses the same principle. The breast is compressed to give a more even thickness of tissue for the X-ray beam to penetrate.

Start at the gas-filled rectum because it is easier to find than the caecum. Follow the line of gas in the colon around to the caecum. Note that it is called gas and not air. Air has a specific composition, and is present in the atmosphere and in the airways.

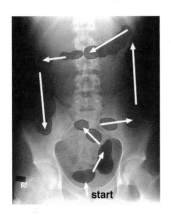

**Fig.** 2.3 Looking at the abdominal gas pattern.

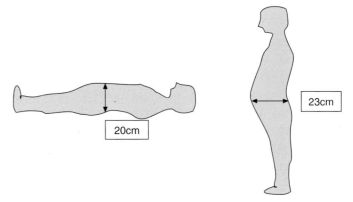

**Fig.** 2.1 Supine and erect abdomen.

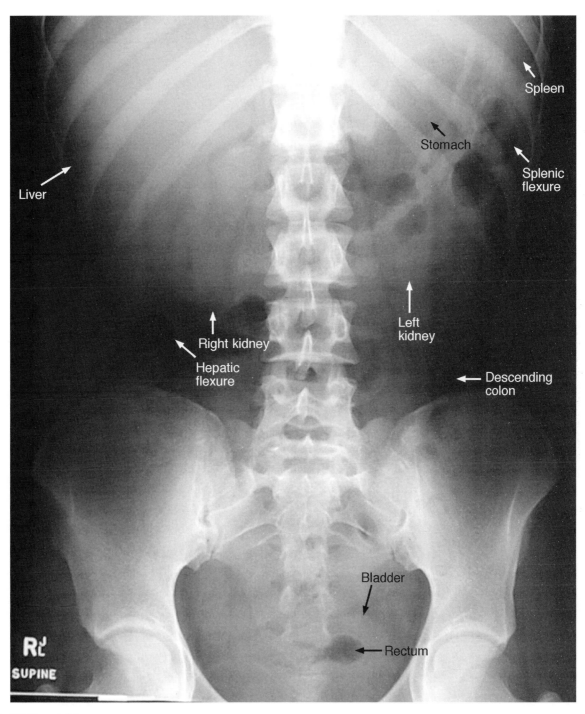

**Fig. 2.2** Normal abdomen.

## What to look for (gas pattern)

### Opacity:

- fluid levels. Three or more fluid levels greater than 2.5 cm in length and in dilated small bowel (greater than 2.5 cm diameter) are abnormal.

### Radiolucency:

- gas. This is normally only seen in the lumen of the stomach, small intestine, and colon. Explain any abnormal quantity of gas in these hollow organs, or gas outside of the lumen of these structures; e.g. pneumoperitoneum, gas in the lumen of the biliary tree or urinary bladder, gas in the wall of the GIT or of the gall bladder.

### Distortion or displacement:

- Check that the stomach, small intestine, and colon are in their normal position. If not, what is displacing them?
- Are they of normal size? The normal maximum diameter of the small intestine is 2.5 cm; of the large intestine, 5 cm; and of the caecum, 9 cm.

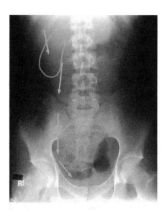

**Fig. 2.4** Looking at the biliary tree and right urinary tract.

## Biliary tree and right urinary tract

Scan the right upper quadrant, the region of the biliary tree, and the right kidney. Look down the line of the right ureter for calcification. The ureter passes near the tips of the lumbar transverse processes, crosses the sacroiliac joint, down to the ischial spine, and then passes medially to join the bladder.

## What to look for

### Opacity:

- gallstone
- renal calculus
- ureteric calculus

### Radiolucency:

- gas in the biliary tree

### Distortion or displacement:

- Check kidney size and shape.
- Look for an absent kidney.
- Look for a pelvic kidney.

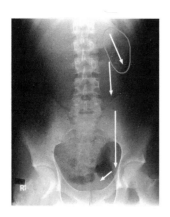

**Fig. 2.5** Looking at the left urinary tract.

## Left urinary tract

Look over to the left kidney, check for renal calculi, and then follow the path of the ureter to the bladder.

## What to look for (left urinary tract)

*Opacity:*

- renal, ureteric, or bladder calculi

*Distortion or displacement:*

- Check kidney size and shape.
- Look for an absent kidney.
- Look for a pelvic kidney.

## Bones—pelvis, vertebral column, and ribs

Start at the right ilium and look around the pelvis, noting the hips and sacroiliac joints. Look at the sacrum, vertebral bodies, and intervertebral disc spaces and lastly glance at the lower ribs.

## What to look for

*Opacity:*

- metastatic deposit—sclerotic deposits are usually from breast and prostate cancer
- degenerative disease of the spine with osteophyte formation
- Paget's disease

*Radiolucency:*

- Most bone metastases are destructive and therefore lucent.

*Distortion:*

- Look for scoliosis.
- Look for expansion of the bones from Paget's disease.

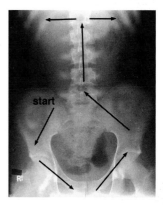

**Fig. 2.6** Looking at the bones.

## Soft tissues

1. *Liver*—look at the size. It should not extend below the level of the ribs in a supine film and with a normal inspiration. This is the same criterion as is used clinically to detect hepatomegaly.

2. *Spleen*—the lower pole of the spleen does not normally extend much below the rib cage. Ultrasound is a better method of detecting hepatosplenomegaly. It can also demonstrate ascites.

3. *Right and left kidney regions*—the left kidney is normally a centimetre or two higher than the right. The liver causes the right hemidiaphragm to be higher and the right kidney to be lower than the left. The presence or absence of the outline of the psoas muscle is not a reliable indicator of the presence or absence of disease.

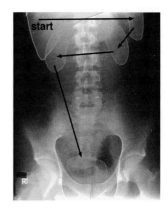

**Fig. 2.7** Looking at the soft tissues.

4. *Pelvis*—the outline of the bladder is usually visible. Check that there are no other soft-tissue masses in the pelvis.

## What to look for

### Opacity:

- calcified granulomas, arteries, lymph nodes

### Radiolucency:

- gas outside the GIT

### Distortion or displacement:

- Check the size and position of liver, spleen, kidneys, bladder.

## The common and important abnormalities of the AXR

### Fluid levels and dilated loops

Both are associated with obstruction and paralytic ileus, but can occur with other diseases.

### Fluid levels

Three fluid levels up to 2.5 cm long can be a normal finding, but longer or more numerous levels mean:

1. *Mechanical obstruction* distal to the fluid levels:

- It can occur at any level of the GIT but most often involves the small intestine.
- The commonest cause is adhesions from previous surgery. Other causes include hernia, tumour, and volvulus.
- If a mechanical obstruction is subacute, i.e. has been present for days or even weeks, most of the gas will have been absorbed, leaving only a small quantity of gas and hence only small fluid levels in a dilated, fluid-filled bowel.
- If the colon is obstructed, the appearance depends on whether the ileocaecal valve is competent. If it is, then only the proximal colon will be distended and not the small intestine.
- Distal to the obstruction, the peristalsis continues and empties the contents of the lumen so the distal bowel is not seen. It is indistinguishable from the surrounding soft tissues.

If a mechanical obstruction is suspected three facts need to be determined so that appropriate treatment can commence, i.e.:

(1) confirm or exclude an obstruction;

(2) identify the site, cause, and severity;

(3) confirm or exclude strangulation (ischaemic bowel).

An abdominal X-ray does not usually provide all this information. A contrast, small-bowel follow-through with barium or iodinated contrast, or a CT study, may be needed.

2. *Paralytic ileus*

A paralytic ileus occurs when the peristalsis stops. Causes include:

- peritonitis;
- postoperative;
- metabolic disturbances;
- local inflammation such as pancreatitis and appendicitis;
- ischaemia of the intestine;
- toxic colon.

The fluid levels and dilated loops may affect all or only part of the intestine.

3. *Gastroenteritis*

With gastroenteritis, fluid levels can be present in the colon as well as in the small intestine.

### Dilated loops

These are caused by:

- mechanical obstruction;
- paralytic ileus;
- hypotonic colon. The loops lose their tone with age.

## Pneumoperitoneum

- This is visible in the supine film if there is a large quantity of free gas.
- As little as 2 ml can be seen under the diaphragm in an erect CXR.
- A cause must be found. Causes include: following laparotomy or laparoscopy; perforated *hollow* viscus, usually a peptic ulcer or a colonic diverticulum; penetrating injury.

## Sick bowel

It is hard to find an elegant term for intestine that appears unwell. The bowel can be the victim of a number of diseases. However, it is a specialized organ and can only react in a limited way no matter what the pathology. Attacks by infection, inflammatory bowel disease, ischaemia (both arterial and venous), radiotherapy, drugs, toxins, and obstruction can all give dilated bowel loops with thickening of the wall. The astute student will ask, 'How can you say if the wall is thick? The gas or barium only shows the lumen.' True. But there are a few tricks. The width of two wall thicknesses can be measured when two loops lie alongside each other. If the wall is oedematous it bulges into the lumen with an appearance like thumbprinting. The valvulae conniventes (plicae circulares, permanent transverse folds of the luminal surface of the small intestine) will appear thickened, as will the folds of the colon.

> ### *Hint*
> Only 75% of cases of intestinal obstruction are diagnosed on an AXR. The others have a non-specific abdominal gas pattern or loops filled with fluid and no gas, the result being that there are no fluid levels.

## Calcification

1. It is important to detect its presence in the *urinary tract*.

2. It is often an incidental finding when seen in the *gall bladder*. If gallstones are suspected, an ultrasound should be ordered.

3. It occurs in lots of places:
   - in the walls of arteries—the aorta, iliac, and splenic arteries are most often affected;
   - in mesenteric lymph nodes in older people—probably the result of ingested TB in unpasteurized milk;
   - calcified granulomas—seen in the liver and spleen from healed infections.

## Summary

At the end of the day, the abdominal X-ray is useful for confirming or excluding the presence of GI obstruction, pneumoperitoneum, sick bowel, and renal tract calcification. It contributes information when the abdominal pain is severe but is of little use with mild or moderate pain. (It is probably ordered too often.)

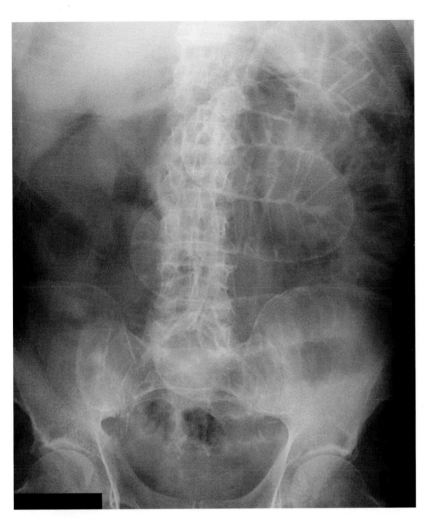

**Fig. 2.8** This is an important film because often these patients are quite unwell and the *supine* abdomen is one of the initial radiographs. The *gas pattern* is of dilated bowel loops. The dilatation is of the small intestine, established by the central position of the loops and the valvulae conniventes which extend fully across the lumen. The large bowel also contains gas. This is therefore: (a) a paralytic ileus, or (b) a distal large bowel obstruction with an incompetent ileocaecal valve, or (c) an acute small bowel obstruction with not enough time for peristalsis to empty the colon. Why is the central loop so well seen? The outside as well as the inside of the wall is clearly visible. The outside wall is only seen because there is gas in the peritoneal cavity, pneumoperitoneum. There has been a perforation and this has caused a paralytic ileus. The *biliary tree* and *right urinary tract*, *left urinary tract*, *bones*, and *soft tissues* add no more information.

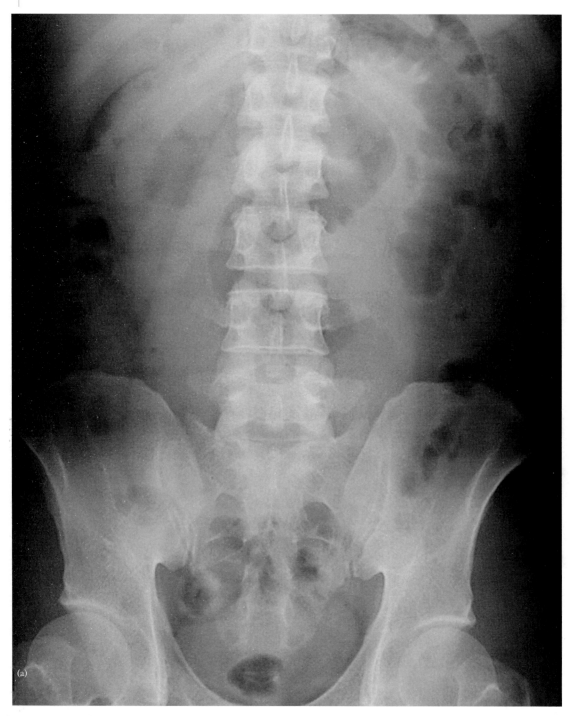

**Figs 2.9** (a) Supine, (b) erect. The fluid levels are immediately obvious in the erect film, but let's approach it in a systematic way. *Gas* can be seen in the colon from the rectum back to the caecum. The stomach bubble is barely visible. That leaves several loops with fluid levels to be explained. They must be small intestine, being centrally placed and with a few valvulae conniventes. The loops are dilated, 3 cm wide, and are probably ileum as the valvulae conniventes are less pronounced here than in the jejunum. By comparison, if the large bowel was obstructed it would show as a few peripheral loops, often over 5 cm in diameter, containing faeces and showing a haustral (scalloped) pattern. Folds in the mucosa of the colon do not extend completely across the lumen. No sign of *calcification in the biliary tree* or *urinary tract*. The *bones* and *soft tissues* are normal. We would be looking for evidence of a cause of small bowel obstruction (SBO): a hernia, surgical clips, or any other signs of surgery.

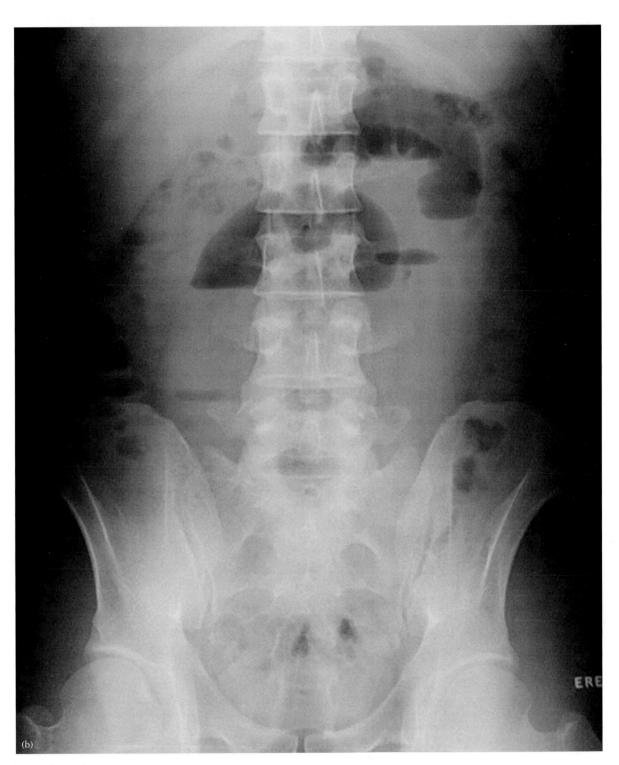

(b)

ERE

**Figs 2.9** *Continued*

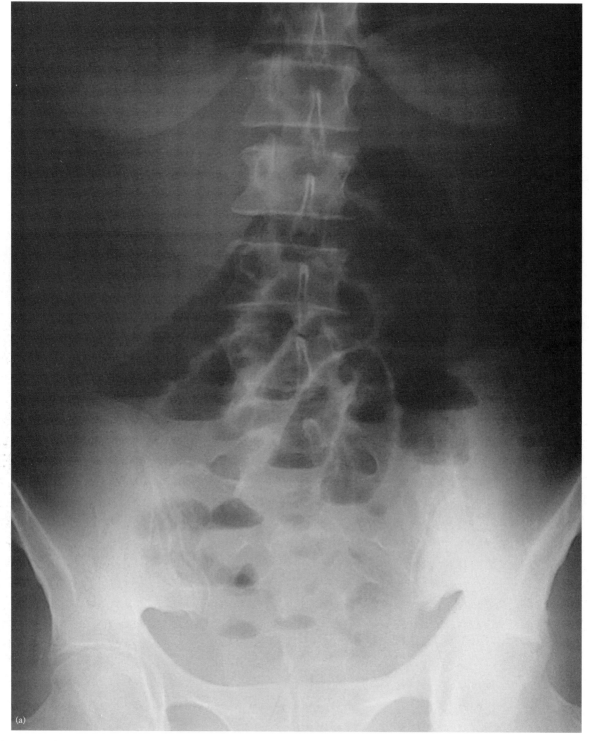

**Figs 2.10** (a), (b) Two images 4 days apart. Both are erect views. Initially the *gas pattern* gives clear evidence of a small bowel obstruction, central loops, and fluid levels. If the obstruction continues it becomes *subacute*; the gas is absorbed and the fluid-filled and dilated loops of small intestine may not be seen. Small quantities of gas remain but are separated by the valvulae conniventes giving the likeness of a string of beads, a subtle but important sign. If the gas has all been absorbed there will be no fluid levels. In this case, to confirm or exclude an obstruction a CT, or contrast swallow and follow-through would be needed. The *biliary tree* and *right urinary tract, left urinary tract, bones*, and *soft tissues* add no more information. A nasogastric tube has been inserted.

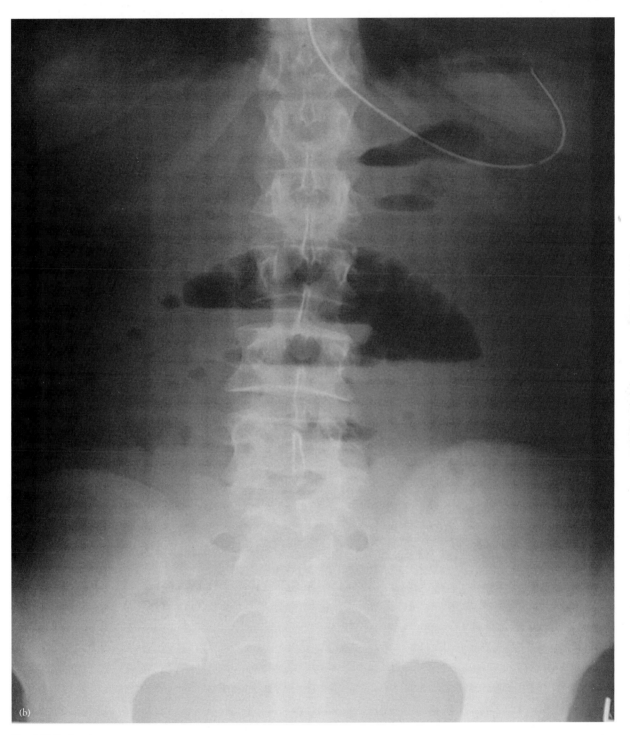

(b)

**Figs 2.10** *Continued*

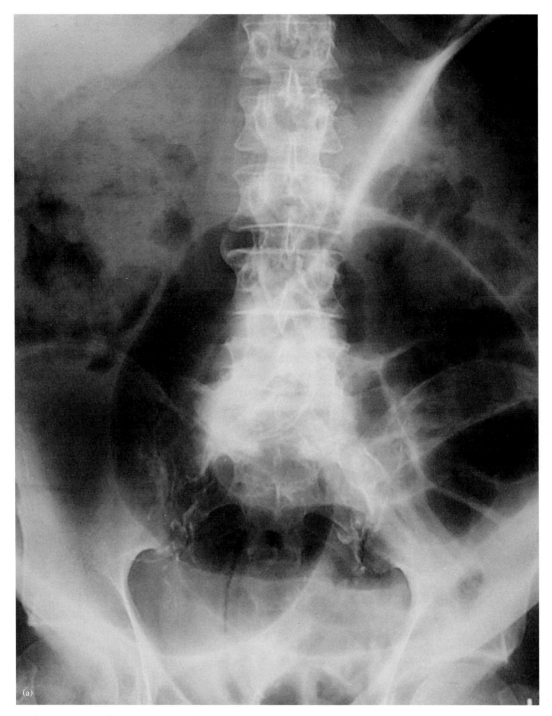

(a)

**Figs** 2.11 (a), (b) Several loops of the intestine are markedly dilated, a central loop with *gas* and other loops with faeces. The dilatation is of the large bowel. If it was a paralytic ileus the small intestine would be involved as well. It must be a type of mechanical obstruction of the colon; a distal large bowel obstruction or a volvulus of the caecum or sigmoid colon. These can be difficult to differentiate. Why not stop guessing and introduce some barium into the rectum to be sure. The *biliary tree* and *right urinary tract*, *left urinary tract*, *bones*, and *soft tissues* add no more information. The barium tapers to a stop at the twist in the sigmoid. Must be a sigmoid volvulus.

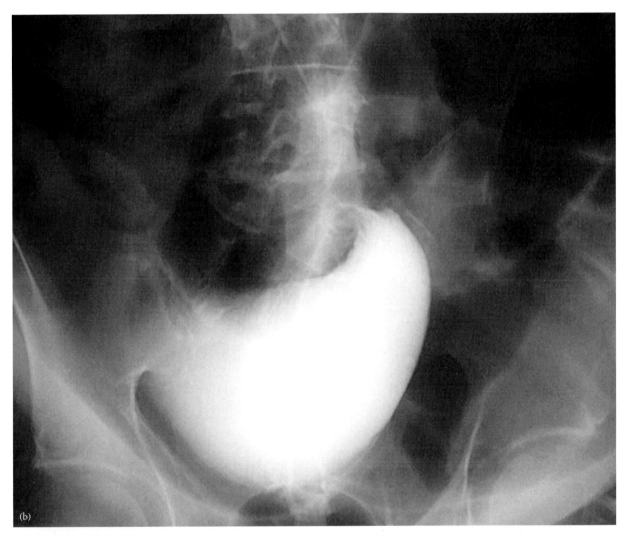

(b)

**Figs 2.11** *Continued*

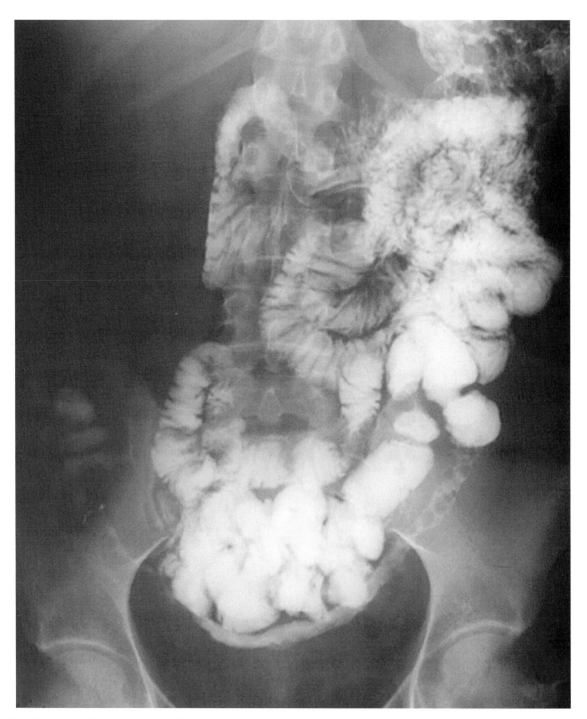

**Fig. 2.12** Barium is used as contrast in a small bowel study to detect inflammatory disease such as Crohn's disease. Here is a long stricture of the terminal ileum. The cobblestone appearance reflects the ulceration and inflammation of the wall. Near the gas-filled caecum the contrast in the lumen is at a considerable distance from the adjacent small bowel loops. This is because of an inflammatory mass, which would be better demonstrated by CT or ultrasound.

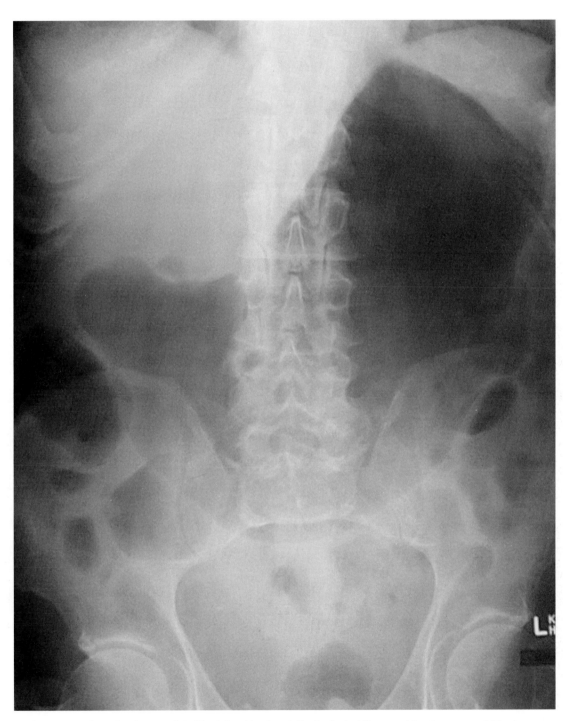

**Fig. 2.13** The *gas pattern* shows that the stomach is dilated. Searching for calcification in the *biliary tree*, *right urinary tract*, and *left urinary tract* reveals calcification in the pelvis. It is probably caused by phleboliths but is difficult to say at times. The *bones* and *soft tissues* are normal. Acute gastric dilatation is a medical emergency and needs prompt decompression with a nasogastric tube. It occurs as a postoperative complication and with diabetic ketoacidosis, trauma, pancreatitis, and hypokalaemia.

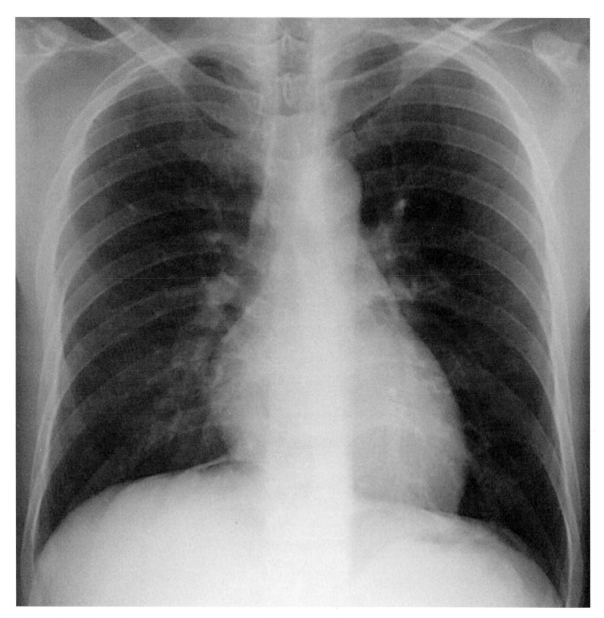

**Fig. 2.14** A few millilitres of gas in the peritoneal cavity can be difficult to see. The best way is with a CXR after remaining erect for 10 min. This may be a small pneumoperitoneum at the right cardiophrenic angle. Check with another view or a CT if necessary. If you strongly suspected a perforated ulcer and the CXR and AXR showed no signs of pneumoperitoneum could you exclude the diagnosis? No. Only 75% of perforations have evidence of pneumoperitoneum.

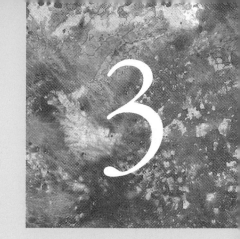

# 3

# Skeletal radiology: trauma

- Skeletal X-rays in trauma:
  How to look for abnormalities
  Where to look
  Rules for trauma imaging
  Complications of fractures that are visible on X-rays

- How to look at:
  The shoulder
  The elbow
  The wrist
  The hip
  The knee
  The ankle
  The foot

# Skeletal radiology: trauma

The main focus and objectives of this chapter are to help the reader become competent in interpreting X-rays of the peripheral skeleton, learning:

(1) normal radiological anatomy;

(2) a system for looking at plain radiographs, both in cases of trauma and where there is no trauma:

    (a) where to look:

        (i) perceptual flow

        (ii) important sites

    (b) what to look for:

        (i) abnormal density

        (ii) abnormal radiolucency

        (iii) distortion or displacement of a normal structure;

(3) how to interpret the abnormalities;

(4) features of several diseases by:

    (a) recognizing the abnormality

    (b) describing it in generic terms

    (c) giving a specific diagnosis

    (d) or knowing where to go to get that information.

Much of the information is contained in the captions.

## Skeletal X-rays in trauma

### How to look for abnormalities

- Ask for the correct images, e.g. the wrist, or the hand, or the scaphoid; the foot, or the ankle, or the calcaneus.
- Make sure they are the correct films. Check the name. It is good practice to look at the name and side marker and turn the film around the correct way *before* putting it on the viewing box.

### Where to look (perhaps just the white parts and then the black parts)

- Look at the body of each bone and then trace the cortex (white parts).
- Look at the joint space, the invisible articular cartilage (black parts).
- Check the soft tissues. In the lateral views of the elbow and the cervical spine, check the soft tissues first as they give indirect evidence of a fracture.

- Different bones and joints have areas that are more prone to fracture or rupture, and these are the places to search carefully. They are described with the radiographs.

## What to look for in cases of trauma

### Opacity:

- overlapping bone fragments

### Radiolucency:

- fracture line

### Distortion or displacement:

- Look for a bump or step or gap in the cortex.
- Look for a buckle or bowing fracture.
- Look for a collapsed vertebra.
- Look for a subluxation or dislocation. A search for a subluxation will reveal a dislocation, so let us just say to look for a fracture or subluxation
- Look for soft-tissue swelling.

## Rules for trauma imaging

1. Two views, or sometimes more, are required.

2. The joints above and below a fracture must be visualized in cases where they may be involved.

3. Once one injury has been found search for another. When a second has been seen, look for a third.

4. Where there is no fracture there may be significant damage to ligaments or the joint capsule.

5. If there is a fracture, the soft tissues have been damaged. The tendon, neural, and vascular damage is not visible on plain films. Check the distal sensation, movement, and pulses.

6. Look for indirect evidence of a fracture, such as displaced fat pads around the elbow joint.

7. Stress views are useful—particularly for the joints of the thumb, fingers, and ankle and the acromioclavicular and scapholunate joints. A force is applied and an X-ray taken to see if subluxation is produced, indicating rupture or strain of the capsule and ligaments of the joint.

8. For a foreign body, X-ray before *and after* removal. Metallic and glass fragments should be visible. Perhaps use a magnifying glass to look for tiny glass fragments.

9. Radiolucent foreign bodies such as wood splinters may be seen and localized with ultrasound.

10. Bone pain in someone with normal bones who has been involved in unaccustomed activity, or in a person with osteopenic bones with normal activity, may be caused by a stress fracture. Often the X-ray is normal. A radionuclear scan will demonstrate it.

11. If the X-rays come back to you without a report there will be instances when you will be unsure if a fracture or subluxation is present or not; in other words the action threshold or the exclusion threshold has not been passed (see Chapter 15). Don't worry. Living with uncertainty is what medicine is all about. There are several options:

    • postpone the decision—put on a plaster and review the next day, or in 7–10 days for a suspected scaphoid fracture;

    • get some more information;

    • order another view;

    • ask a colleague, a senior, or a radiologist;

    • look up a book such as the *Atlas of normal roentgen variants that may simulate disease* (Keats 1996) or *An atlas of normal developmental roentgen anatomy* (Keats and Smith 1988);

    • check a reference book such as *Orthopedic radiology* (Greenspan 1996) or *Accident and emergency radiology, a survival guide* (Raby *et al*.1995);

    • use another modality, CT, MRI, or RNS;

    • (rarely) X-ray the other side for comparison.

12. As with all medical imaging, abnormalities in trauma radiographs are of three types:

    • an opacity

    • a radiolucency

    • distortion or displacement of a normal structure.

Anyone who only looks for a radiolucency (fracture line) is courting disaster.

It is best to learn a few of the common descriptors of fractures so that you can describe them over the phone, the orthopaedic people may then treat you with respect.

useful descriptors are: *transverse*, *oblique*, *spiral*, *buckle*, *greenstick*;

*closed*: intact skin;

*open*: connected to the atmosphere;

*comminuted*: more than two fragments, the smaller fragments may have impaired perfusion;

*avulsion*: when the tensile strength of the ligament or tendon is greater than that of the bone;

*impacted*: occurs in the neck of the femur and the neck of the humerus;

*compression* or *wedge*: fracture of a vertebra: results from axial loading or a flexion injury;

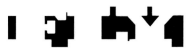

Fig. 3.1 Take this simple test. Look at the black parts and you won't see the white word.

*alignment*: involves the *displacement, angulation, rotation,* and *overriding* or *distraction of the fragments*—if the alignment is good after a fracture is reduced it means that the bone ends are apposed (no overriding or distraction), that there is no displacement to the front or back or to either side, no angulation of the distal fragment relative to the proximal, and no rotation;

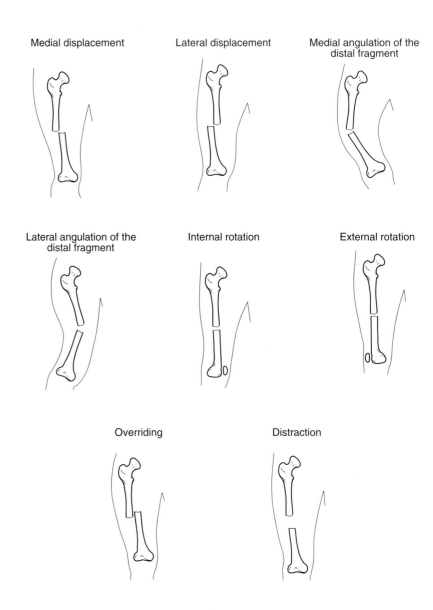

Fig. 3.2 Alignment of fractures.

*Salter–Harris types* I–V describe fractures of the epiphyseal plate of growing bones.

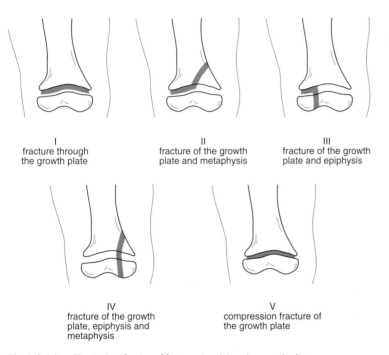

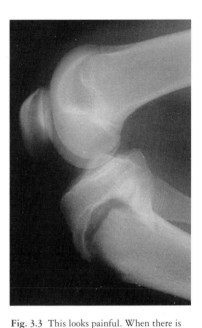

**Fig. 3.3** This looks painful. When there is trauma the weakest link gives way. In this 15-year-old male it is the growth plate (the physis or epiphyseal line). This is a Salter–Harris type II fracture. When fractures involve the growth plate the injuries can be separated into five groups which reflect the severity, likelihood of complications, and prognosis. Complications are mainly arrest of growth in part of the physis (giving angulation) or all of the physis with fusion of the epiphysis to the metaphysis (giving shortening). It can be a problem if one limb becomes shorter than the other or, in this case, if the tibia does not grow as much as the fibula.

**Fig. 3.4** Salter–Harris classification of fractures involving the growth plate.

## Complications of fractures that are visible on X-rays

These include:

- mal-union—healing in an unacceptable position;

- delayed union—not united in 6 months;

- non-union—fails to unite and no evidence that union is likely to occur;

- osteoarthrosis from involvement of the joint initially or from mal-union and consequent distortion of the lines of force that act on the joint;

- disuse osteoporosis;

- infection—*acute* osteomyelitis exhibits bone destruction and periostial reaction on an X-ray—*chronic* osteomyelitis shows as thick, sclerotic (footnote 7) (white) bone;

- osteonecrosis, typically of the proximal bone fragment of the scaphoid where it complicates 10% of fractures. May take 6 months to become apparent. The proximal fragment will be sclerotic.

---

7  Hardening or induration from the Greek *sklerosis*. Used also for hardening of the blood vessels, atherosclerosis, and in the nervous system where the hardening takes the form of deposition of connective tissue e.g. multiple sclerosis.

How to look at

## The shoulder

*Where to look*

- Look at the humerus, scapula, and clavicle and then trace the cortex (white parts).
- Look at the joint spaces of the glenohumeral and acromioclavicular joints (black parts).
- Look at the soft tissues.

## What to look for

*Opacity:*

- impacted fracture of the surgical neck of the humerus

*Radiolucency:*

- fracture line of the neck or greater tuberosity of the humerus; less commonly, the scapula or distal clavicle

*Distortion or displacement:*

- In the lateral film follow the shaft of the humerus up to the head and it will be projected over the glenoid, at the junction of the three arms of a 'Y'— these being the coracoid process, the acromion, and the body of the scapula. See that the end of the clavicle is aligned with the acromion.

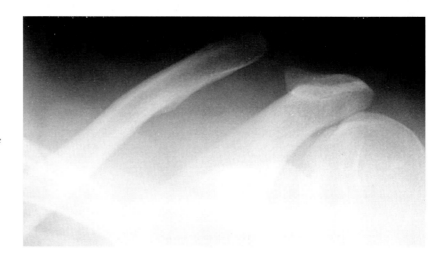

**Fig. 3.5** *Bones*: normal *Joints*: Distortion of the normal acromioclavicular joint with dislocation. Follow the line of the inferior margin of the clavicle. The line should continue along the inferior margin of the acromion without any step. There must be rupture of the acromioclavicular ligament and in this case rupture of the coracoclavicular ligament. Sometimes stress views and comparison views of the other side are helpful in more discrete cases of subluxation with ligamentous sprain.

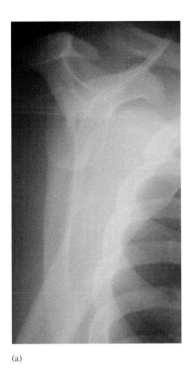

(a)

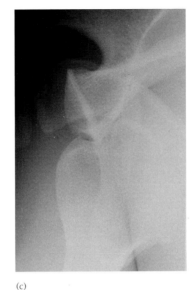

(c)

Figs 3.6 (a)–(d)  A true lateral view of the scapula gives it a 'Y' appearance. The coracoid process points anteriorly and is the direction of the dislocation—95% of dislocations are anterior, 5% posterior. The acromion forms the posterior limb of the 'Y'. A dislocation can be distinguished because the head of the humerus no longer lies in the middle of the 'Y' of the scapula. Follow the shaft of the humerus up to the head. It lies at the centre of the 'Y' in the postreduction film. An anterior dislocation sometimes causes a Hill–Sach's fracture, an indentation of the humeral head, also seen in the postreduction film.

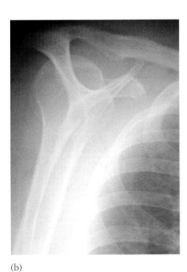

(b)

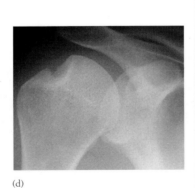

(d)

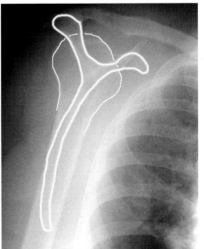

Fig. 3.7  Lateral view of the scapula. It is an oblique view of the *shoulder* because the scapula lies posterolaterally on the chest wall, not posterior.

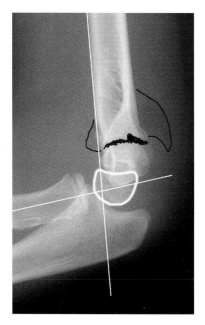

**Fig. 3.8** The elbow with displaced anterior and posterior fat pads and a supracondylar fracture. The capitellum is displaced posteriorly.

## The elbow

### Where to look

- Look at the soft tissues first for the 'fat pad sign'.
- Look at the humerus, ulna, and radius and then trace the cortex.
- Look at the articular cartilage (black parts).

## What to look for

### Radiolucency:

- fracture line

### Distortion or displacement:

- A displaced fat pad indicates fluid in the elbow **joint**. The fluid, usually blood, causes this appearance because the fat pads lie outside the synovium and joint capsule. Normally the anterior fat pad lies along the anterior surface of the humerus and the posterior fat pad occupies the olecranon fossa, out of sight.
- Check for a buckle or step in the cortex.
- Check for an incongruity of articular surfaces.
- The anterior humeral line and the line of the long axis of the radius should each pass through the middle third of the capitellum.

**Figs 3.9** (a), (b)  The first glance at the lateral film reveals displaced fat pads, anteriorly and posteriorly. It is then only a matter of finding the fracture. *Bones*: A check of the *bones* reveals the fracture line. It is superior to the condyles (the trochlea and capitellum) and is therefore called a supracondylar fracture. Next, look for any distortion or displacement. The key feature is the capitellum (called the *capitulum* in anatomy books) in the lateral view. In this instance the distal humerus, including the capitellum, is displaced posteriorly. *Joint*: There is no subluxation.

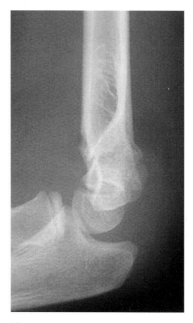

(a)

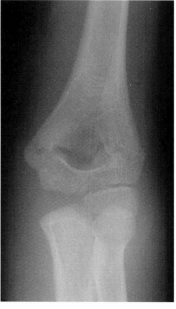

(b)

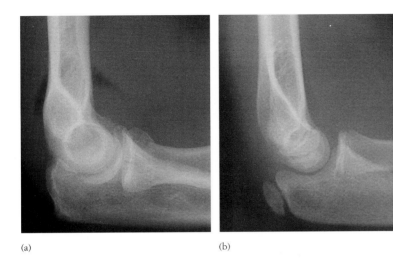

(a)　　　　　　　　(b)

**Figs 3.10** (a) Post-trauma, (b) Normal. The abnormal anterior fat pad is bowed forwards to adopt the shape of a rose thorn. The posterior fat pad is visible. *Bones*: The cause of the haemarthrosis is often a fracture of the radial head. It may need several views to demonstrate it, seen here as a disruption of the cortex. The anterior humeral line and the line of the longitudinal axis of the radius pass through the middle one-third of the capitellum. *Joint*: No subluxation.

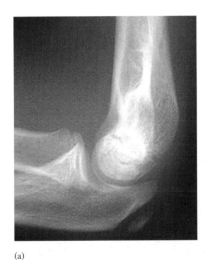

(a)

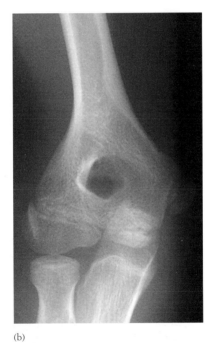

(b)

**Figs 3.11** (a), (b) Normal ossification centres of the elbow. Look for the medial and lateral epicondyles (footnote 8). The *l*ateral ossifies *l*ast, meaning that if it is visible the medial one must be there. If the medial epicondyle cannot be seen, is it avulsed and pulled into the elbow joint? The olecranon epiphysis is displayed in the lateral view

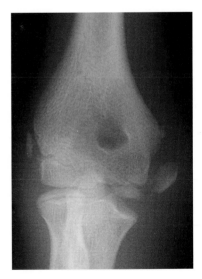

**Fig. 3.12** 15-year-old male. *Bones*: No abnormal opacity. No fracture line seen. But there is displacement of the medial epicondyle, an avulsion fracture, usually associated with elbow dislocation. *Joint*: No subluxation—the dislocation has reduced.

---

8　Epi- a prefix meaning 'on', 'above', or 'near'.

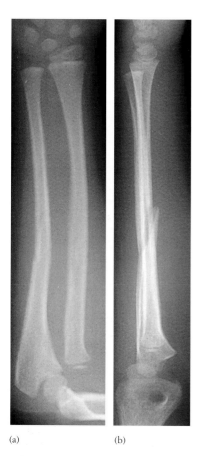

(a)          (b)

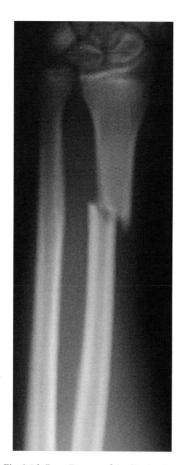

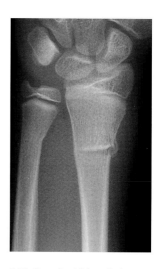

**Fig. 3.15** *Bones*: In children the bones are more malleable and a fracture can be a greenstick fracture such as this, with a fracture of one cortex, a bowing fracture where the shaft is bowed, or a buckle fracture, a buckle of the cortex. This is an image where it is easy to see that something is wrong. Remember to look for the second abnormality. There is a greenstick fracture of the distal radius and just that bit of angulation to indicate a buckle fracture of the ulna. *Joints*: normal.

**Figs 3.13** (a), (b) *Bones*: There is a fracture of the ulna. *Joints*: The radius is dislocated. These films demonstrate two rules: (1) with a fracture of a bone the joints above and below often need to be visualized; (2) the line of the axis of the radius should pass through the middle third of the capitellum. This is called a Monteggia fracture, a fracture of the ulna and dislocation of the proximal radius. A Galeazzi fracture is less common and is a fracture of the distal radius with a subluxation or dislocation of the distal radioulnar joint. How does one remember which is which. If the examiner or orthopaedic surgeon asks 'What fracture is this?' say 'UM…' and that is the clue; *U*lna fracture = *M*onteggia.

**Fig. 3.14** *Bones*: Fracture of the distal radius with shortening. Look for the second fracture, the ulna styloid. *Joints*: Find the displacement of normal structures, subluxation of the distal radioulnar joint. The line of force has passed through these three structures. This is a Galeazzi fracture/subluxation.

## The wrist

### Where to look

- Look at the radius, ulna, carpal bones, and metacarpals and then trace the cortex (white parts).
- Look at the joints (black parts).
- Look at the soft tissues.

## What to look for

### Opacity:

- overlapping bone fragments

### Radiolucency:

- fracture line, particularly of the scaphoid or radius

### Distortion or displacement:

- The bony articular surfaces should be parallel, separated only by 2 mm of the radiolucent articular cartilage.
- Check the position of the distal ulna relative to the radius.
- Consider that the lunate is the halfback or quarterback of the carpal bone team. Check that all adjacent bones are correctly related to it, no widening of the scapholunate distance (2 mm) indicating a rupture of the ligament. On the lateral view, the radius, lunate, and capitate should be aligned.

### Hint

When examining the X-ray following reduction of the fracture fragments, look both at the alignment of the bones and then at the shape of the plaster cast on the X-ray to admire the moulding. The aim is to achieve not only an anatomical reduction but also moulding of the cast to hold the position.

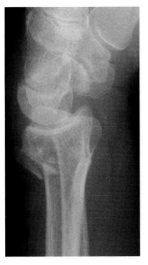

(a)

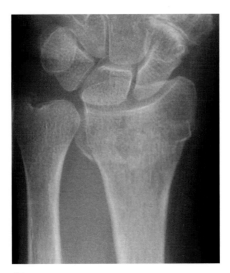

(b)

Figs 3.16 (a), (b) Falling on an outstretched hand can produce a number of injuries, including fractures of the scaphoid, distal radius, and a supracondylar fracture of the humerus. Knowing the mechanism of injury is important as it leads to understanding and directs attention to likely sites of injury. *Bones*: The fracture lines and distortion are not difficult to see. A Colles' (or Pouteau) fracture is one of the distal radius, usually with dorsal angulation and dorsal displacement of the distal fragment. There is often an accompanying fracture of the ulna styloid. This fracture does not have the dorsal displacement to fit the description, only the angulation and the fracture of the ulna styloid. In any case, there are varying interpretations of what makes a Colles' fracture. It may be better to describe the fracture rather than use an eponym. No other injury was seen when looking for the third abnormality, but the bones of the wrist have thinned cortex and are probably osteoporotic. *Joints*: The scaphotrapezium joint is narrowed because of loss of articular cartilage, and there is subarticular sclerosis. These are the signs of osteoarthrosis

**Figs 3.17** (a), (b) Normal bones of the wrist. (PA view): The bones of the wrist are in order, clockwise or anticlockwise (depending on which wrist) from the scaphoid (footnote 9): lunate, triquetrum, and overlying pisiform; hamate with the hook (arrow); capitate, the largest bone; and the trapezoid and trapezium. (lateral view): In a true lateral a straight line passes through the ulna, radius, lunate, capitate, and metacarpals 2–5.

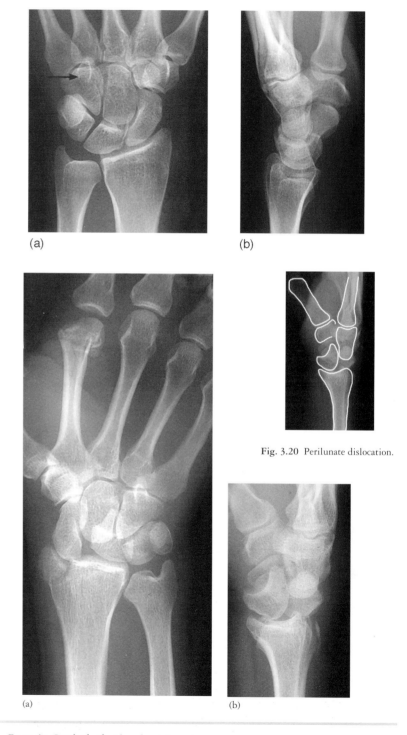

(a)                    (b)

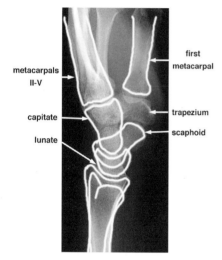

Fig. 3.18 Lateral wrist.

Fig. 3.20 Perilunate dislocation.

**Figs 3.19** (a), (b) *Bones*: In the AP projection the obvious abnormality is a fracture of the radial styloid process. *Joints*: The alignment of the proximal bones of the wrist is distorted. The scapholunate distance is widened, indicating rupture of the scapholunate ligament. Furthermore, the lateral projection indicates that the lunate does not sit normally in the concavity of the radius and that the capitate no longer articulates with the lunate. This is a perilunate dislocation.

*Note*: Don't forget the rule 'once one abnormality is seen, look for the next'. Fracture of the head and neck of the second metacarpal.

(a)                    (b)

9   From the Greek *skaphoeides* = boat shaped.

## Tips and tricks

1. How do I avoid missing a fracture? Examine the patient carefully, and *before ordering the X-ray* decide what you will do if the X-ray comes back normal. Do **not** leave that decision until the time when the X-ray is reported.

   If the chance of a fracture is low, you can accept what appears to be a normal film. If the chance of a fracture is high, you may decide that a normal X-ray will not be an endpoint, the exclusion threshold will not be passed. Further views or opinions, imaging with another modality, or treatment as if a fracture is present may be the way to proceed.

   If you allow the X-ray to be the sole arbiter of whether disease is present you will never develop a high level of clinical judgement. Consider two scenarios:

   (1) cursory history and examination, X-ray requested:
   - fracture demonstrated → treat;
   - no fracture or subluxation demonstrated → reassurance ± bandage ± aspirin;

   (2) history and examination that assesses the probability of fracture, X-ray requested:
   - fracture demonstrated → treat;
   - no fracture or subluxation demonstrated;
   - in a case of low probability of a fracture → reassurance, etc.;
   - in a case of high probability of a fracture → further views or opinions, imaging with another modality, or treatment as if a fracture is present → fewer fractures missed → better clinical judgement as the feedback from the X-rays refines your skill in allocating probability.

2. Use a system to look at X-rays. Go carefully through each area of interest once only.

3. Write your assessment or diagnosis where the radiologist can review it and provide feedback. This will force you to make a decision, help the radiologist appreciate where teaching is needed, and accelerate your learning.

4. Show interesting cases to others. This will improve your perception and if your colleagues do the same will expose you to many good films.

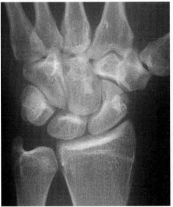 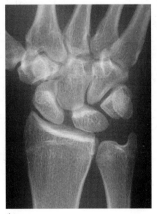

(a)  (b)

**Figs 3.21** (a) Left wrist, (b) Right wrist. Plain X-rays are quite an insensitive test for damage from trauma as the bones are usually the only structures demonstrated. Damage to nerves, arteries, veins, muscles, ligaments, joint capsules, and skin must all be assessed clinically, diagnosed accurately, and treated accordingly. *Bones*: There is a fracture of the distal pole of the left scaphoid. The small opacities in the left scaphoid and capitate bones are incidental findings. It is probably safe to call them bone islands, areas of dense cortical bone which have developed in the medullary cavity for some reason or another which we may never know. *Joints*: Occasionally the appearance of the bones gives indirect evidence of soft-tissue damage. In this case the distance between the right scaphoid and lunate bones is increased to more than the allowable 2 mm. Comparison with the other wrist confirms this finding, which indicates a rupture of the scapholunate ligament, probably requiring surgical repair.

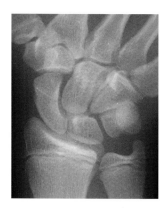

**Fig. 3.22** *Bones*: This fracture of the waist of the scaphoid is important as it can interfere with the blood supply to the proximal end and may cause avascular necrosis. The distal end has a separate artery and does not have this complication. This fracture is not easy to see. If in doubt ask for another view. *Joints*: normal alignment.

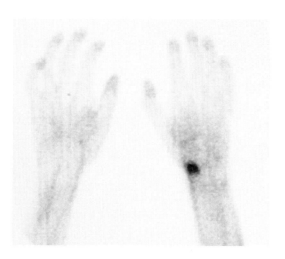

**Fig. 3.23** A suspected fracture of the scaphoid can be immobilized and X-rayed again in 10 days. Alternative methods of demonstrating a fracture are: radionuclear imaging, such as is demonstrated here; MRI; or CT. The isotope is taken up at the site of bone repair. Other causes of increased uptake on a bone scan include arthritis, infection, neoplasm, and Paget's disease.

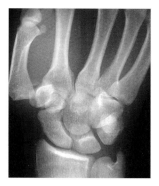

**Fig. 3.24** *Bones*: The abnormal opacity between the bases of the first and second metacarpals is the fragment of the first metacarpal that remains in position. The larger fragment has been dislocated radially and dorsally, the direction determined by the pull of the abductor pollicis longus. This is a Bennett fracture/dislocation of the base of the first metacarpal, involving the articular surface. *Joints*: The joint capsule and the interosseous ligament attaching the bone to the trapezium will be ruptured, making immobilization difficult. Internal fixation with a wire is required.

## Tips and tricks

- To avoid confusion call fingers by their name, not by numbers.

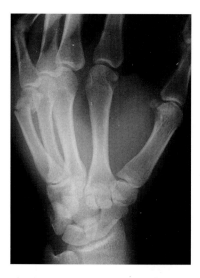

**Fig. 3.25** *Bones*: A common injury from punching a wall out of frustration. The distortion of the alignment caused by this fracture of the neck of the 5th metacarpal is easy to see. As with almost all fractures a check film is required after immobilization. This can indicate the alignment in the frontal and lateral planes but will not disclose any rotation. Rotation is assessed clinically (alignment of the fingernails). *Joints*: normal.

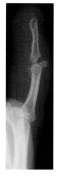

**Fig. 3.26** *Bones*: Perhaps the easiest fracture to understand with regard to the mechanism of injury. An object, usually a ball, hits the tip of the outstretched finger causing flexion of the distal interphalangeal joint. Sometimes an avulsion fracture results, but in 75% of cases the extensor tendon is avulsed with no bone fragment. The deformity, flexion at the distal interphalangeal joint, is called a mallet finger or baseball finger. *Joints*: The fracture line involves the joint surface. The sensitivity of plain X-rays for detecting an avulsion *fracture* is almost 100%. The more important sensitivity of an X-ray detecting the cause of *a mallet finger* (rupture of the tendon *or* avulsion of a bone fragment) is 100%–75% = 25%.

## The hip

### Where to look

- Look at the femur and the pelvis and then trace the cortex (white parts).
- Look at the 'joint spaces' (black parts).
- Look at the soft tissues.

## What to look for

**Opacity:**

- impacted fracture of the neck of the femur

**Radiolucency:**

- fracture line

**Distortion or displacement:**

- In cases of trauma look carefully at the trabecular pattern of the neck of the femur and at the acetabulum, and pubic rami.

In plain X-rays of the hip, the surrounding soft tissues are not a guide to pathology in cases of trauma.

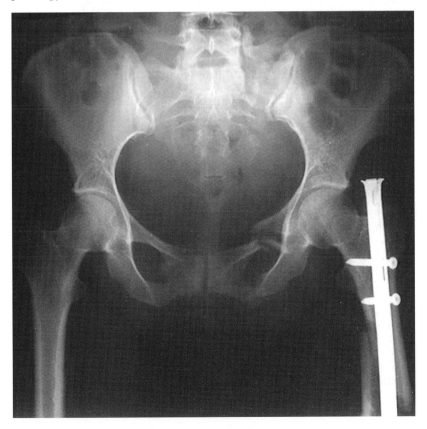

**Fig. 3.27** *Bones*: The fractures of the left superior and inferior pubic rami are easy to see. The second fracture is that of the right pubic bone. The third is of the shaft of the left femur, treated with an intramedullary nail. The pelvis is a bony ring. The pubic rami fractures, with separation of the fragments, may be accompanied by another. The fourth fracture is in the sacrum. The left wing of the sacrum is displaced superiorly to the level of L5. This unstable pelvic fracture is called a Malgaigne fracture. *Joints*: The hips, pubic symphysis, and sacroiliac joints appear intact. Fractures of the pubic bones in males, particularly towards the midline, can tear the membranous urethra. Risk management dictates that, in cases where voluntary voiding is not possible or where blood comes from the urethra, a urethrogram should be performed. It will demonstrate the patency of the lumen so that a catheter may pass safely.

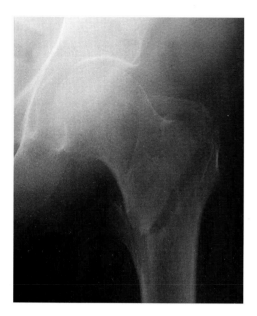

**Fig. 3.28** *Bones*: The fracture line extends from the greater trochanter above, to the lesser trochanter situated below and medially, an intertrochanter fracture. It has the advantage of not interfering significantly with the blood supply to the head of the femur. Internal fixation can therefore be with a compression screw and plate. *Joint*: normal

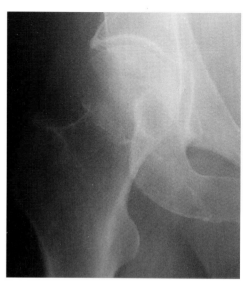

**Fig. 3.29** *Bones*: The opacity is an impacted fracture of the neck of the femur (subcapital position) confirmed by the distortion of the cortex. The blood supply to the head of the femur is compromised and a hemiarthroplasty (femoral head prosthesis) may be required.

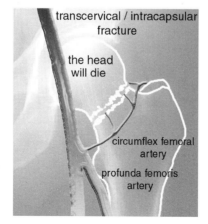

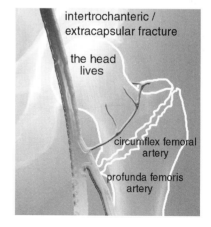

**Fig. 3.30** Blood supply to the head of the femur.

## The knee

*Where to look*

- Look at the femur, patella, tibia, and fibula and then trace the cortex (white parts).
- Look at the joint space (black parts).
- Look at the soft tissues.

## What to look for

*Opacity:*

- include a search for a loose body in the joint

*Radiolucency:*

- look carefully for the fractures of the tibial plateaux and intercondylar eminence. If in doubt ask for oblique views or a CT

*Distortion or displacement:*

In trauma pay attention to:
- alignment of the medial and lateral femoral and tibial condyles;
- alignment of the fibula—on the AP film the highest point of the fibula is near the lateral margin of the tibia;
- distension of the suprapatellar pouch with fluid.

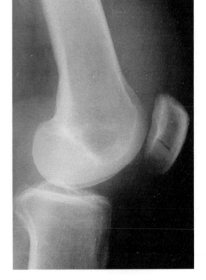

Fig. 3.32 *Bones*: It was difficult to appreciate the fracture of the patella on the frontal projection. The lateral view shows the radiolucency of the fracture line. *Joint*: Above the patella is a distended, blood-filled, suprapatellar pouch pushing the quadriceps tendon anteriorly. This would confirm a clinical finding of haemarthrosis.

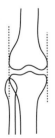

Normal alignment of margins of the femur and tibia and of the apex of the fibula to the lateral margin of the tibia

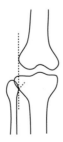

Suspicion of a fracture of the lateral tibial plateau. Check the oblique views. Think of a CT.

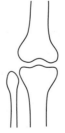

Subluxation of the proximal tibio-fibular joint

Fig. 3.31 Alignment of the medial and lateral femoral and tibial condyles.

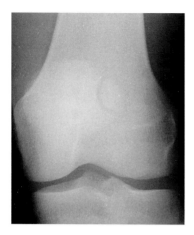

**Fig. 3.33** Bipartite patella, caused by an accessory ossification centre. A normal variant.

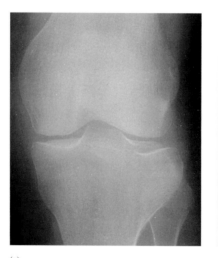

(a)

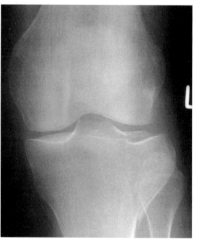

(b)

**Figs 3.34** (a) Initial film, (b) 8 days later. Bumper bar vs. pedestrian. Trauma to the lateral side of the knee. Looking only for a fracture line (a radiolucency) in cases of trauma is fraught with danger. Initially this fracture was missed. Oblique views would help but the information is there: distortion and displacement. *Bones*: The lateral margin of the tibia should align with that of the femur, as on the medial side. Additionally, the apex of the head of the fibula should be at the lateral margin of the tibia. *Joint*: The fracture line involves the joint surface. An X-ray 8 days later demonstrated the fracture more clearly. One of the reasons it was missed was because many knee X-rays after trauma have no bone or joint abnormality. This can lead to an expectation of a normal radiograph. The delay in this diagnosis may not have happened if there was a careful clinical examination, systematic approach to reading the film, no prejudgement of the film, and enough time to diagnose and treat adequately

## The ankle

*Where to look*

- Look at the tibia, fibula, talus, and other visible foot bones, particularly the base of the fifth metatarsal after trauma, and then trace the cortex (white parts).

- Look at the joint spaces (black parts). The ankle is a complex hinge joint but on AP views looks like a mortise and tenon joint, the mortise formed by the tibia and fibula. The width of the joint space should be uniform.

- Check the alignment.

## What to look for

*Opacity:*

- Overlapping fragments or compressed bone.

*Radiolucency:*

- Don't forget to check the neck of the talus and the base of the fifth metatarsal for fractures.

*Distortion or displacement:*

- Check for equal distance around the ankle mortise.

- Estimate whether the width of the distal tibiofibular syndesmosis is normal.

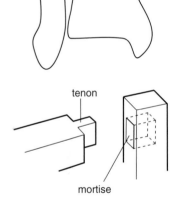

**Fig. 3.35** The ankle mortise. Mortise and tenon joint, useful in manufacture of furniture.

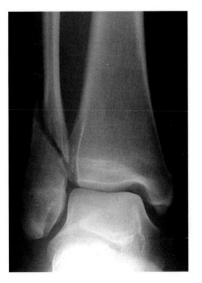

**Fig. 3.36** Fractures of the ankle are complex. If you aim at detecting a fracture or subluxation and turning it over to someone who knows about treatment you can't get into much trouble. Several classifications are available, the best perhaps is that by Weber (1972) because it emphasizes the importance of whether the distal tibiofibular syndesmosis is intact. *Bones*: Spiral fracture of the distal fibula. *Joints*: The syndesmosis is essentially intact (some posterior fibres may be torn). There is probably rupture of the deltoid ligament (medially). This is a Weber type B ankle injury. The fibula fracture is *at* the level of the syndesmosis. In Type A, there is a fracture of the medial malleolus. If there is a fracture of the lateral malleolus it is *below* the level of the syndesmosis. Otherwise there will be a rupture of the lateral collateral ligament. The syndesmosis will be intact. Type C fractures have disruption of the malleolus or deltoid ligament on the medial side, disruption (diastasis) of the distal tibiofibular syndesmosis, and a fracture of the fibula *above* the level of the syndesmosis.

## The foot

### Where to look

- Look at the bones of the midfoot, the metatarsals, and phalanges and then trace the cortex (white parts).
- Look at the joints (black parts). Check the alignment; see that the three joints between the bases of the 1–4 metatarsals align with the two joints between the cuneiforms and the joint between the lateral cuneiform and the cuboid.
- Look at the soft tissues.

## What to look for

### Opacity:

- Sclerotic reaction of healing in a stress fracture

### Radiolucency:

- Fracture line

### Distortion or displacement:

- A fracture or subluxation of the tarsometatarsal joint must be searched for because it is easily missed. It can result from a relatively minor injury such as walking in a pothole, and also occurs with major trauma where it may be overlooked because attention is diverted to an ankle injury.

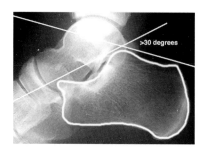

**Fig. 3.38** Boehler's angle of the calcaneus.

**Fig. 3.37** *Bones*: This radiograph demonstrates the three appearances of a fracture: opacity, radiolucency, and distortion of the cortex. *Joint*: The subtalar joint is involved. A fracture of the calcaneus usually occurs because of landing on the feet when falling from a height. It obtained the colourful name of 'lover's fracture' as it was sustained by the fleeing party in a leap from the window as the spouse arrived home. Is this an urban myth? Was it a first-floor apartment? We need to know three things: does the fracture involve the subtalar joint; is it bilateral because of the mechanism of injury; and is there an axial-loading, compression fracture of the lumbar spine? The degree of flattening of the calcaneus can be assessed by Boehler's angle. This is the angle formed when the lines from the posterosuperior and the anterosuperior margins of the calcaneus meet at the highest point of the tip of the posterior facet of the subtalar joint. Normally it should be >30°.

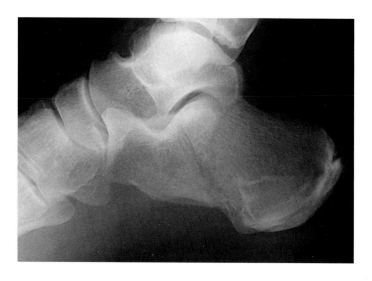

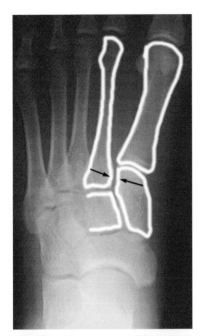

**Fig. 3.39** Normal width for this part of the tarsometatarsal (Lisfranc) joint.

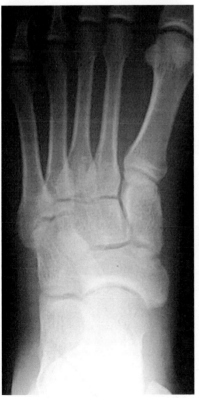

AP view

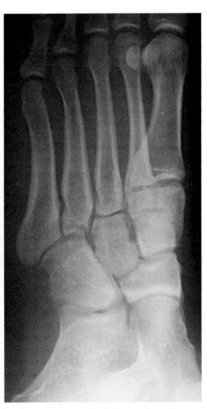

Oblique

**Fig. 3.40** The foot arches in two planes: AP and coronal. One bone is often superimposed on another. Order extra views if needed. CT is sometimes necessary to define the anatomy. The medial and lateral borders of the bases of the 1st–3rd metatarsals must align with the edges of the medial, intermediate, and lateral cuneiform bones. Check the alignment of the 4th and 5th metatarsals with the cuboid.

**Fig. 3.41** Lisfranc fracture/subluxation of the tarsometatarsal joint is often disclosed by the widening here at the base of the 2nd metatarsal and the medial cuneiform.

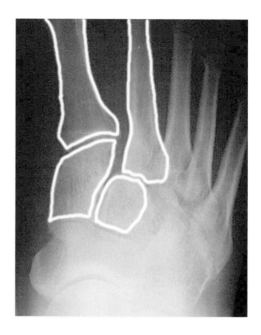

**Fig. 3.42** *Bones*: Initially no fracture seen. *Joints*: In the right foot the medial edge of the 2nd metatarsal does not correctly align with the medial edge of the intermediate cuneiform. Opacities, avulsed bone fragments, lie in the widened space between the medial aspect of the base of the 2nd metatarsal and the medial cuneiform. This is a fracture/subluxation of the tarsometatarsal joint, a Lisfranc fracture/subluxation. This radiograph has been selected to demonstrate the principle of how to detect the abnormality. It is not the most obvious example. If the more subtle changes are appreciated, the gross abnormalities should be no problem.

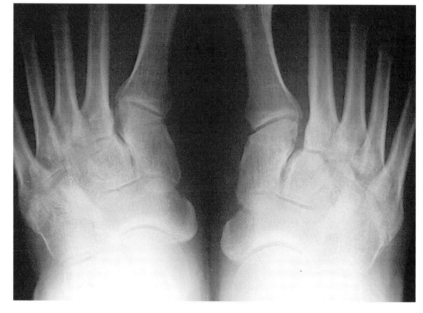

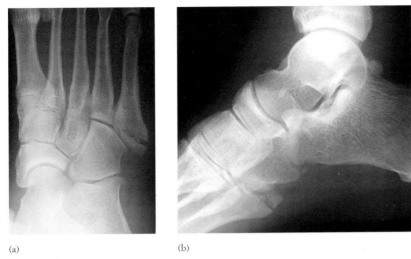

(a)                          (b)

**Figs 3.43** (a), (b) *Bones*: Avulsion fracture of the base of the 5th metatarsal, the result of an inversion injury. The tendon of peroneus brevis is obviously stronger than the bone (greater *tensile* strength). *Joints*: normal. Accessory ossification centres are often seen around the ankle joint. Two are visible here. They are well corticated and in documented positions. Consult a book of 'Normal variants' when in doubt.

**Fig. 3.44** The cortex contributes most of the opacity of the bone to X-rays, and that is because it contains calcium which has a relatively high atomic number (20), meaning 20 electrons in orbit to deflect the X-ray photons. Most of the radio-opacity of what looks like the medullary cavity is caused by the dense cortex at the front and back. *Bones*: The fracture has occurred in a weakened part of the humerus where the cortex is eroded and thinned and replaced by soft tissue that does not contain calcium. It is a process that started in the medullary cavity and is therefore probably blood-borne. This is a metastatic deposit of breast carcinoma. Fracture in abnormal bone is called a pathological fracture. *Joints*: normal. *Soft tissues*: The tumour appears to be extending beyond the cortex.

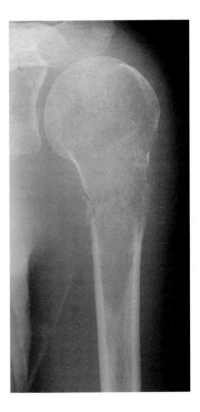

**Fig. 3.45** It takes real clinical skill to detect a case of non-accidental injury (NAI) and on the other hand to avoid having too high an index of suspicion which will cause a lot of work and ill-feeling. Radiological features of NAI include those seen here:

- Fractures of various ages are seen in the long bones, demonstrated by radiolucent lines, callus formation, and periosteal reaction (proliferation of the periosteum with calcification, seen here around the shaft of the right femur).
- Metaphyseal fractures are characteristic but not as common as those in the shaft. The right femoral and tibial metaphyses are fractured.

*Notes*:

- Non-accidental injury is only one aspect of child abuse (mental and physical). Mental abuse increases with age so that teenagers may have twice the risk of mental and physical abuse as infants and young children under 3 years of age (McMahon *et al.* 1995). The young children are more likely to have fractures as a result of abuse.
- Suspicious fractures include those of the posterior ribs from grabbing and squeezing the child, skull fractures in children under 2 years of age, metaphyseal fractures, and fractures of various ages in the long bones.
- Fractures occur in up to 50% of the cases of non-accidental injury. The explanation of the cause may be implausible. Absence of fractures does not exclude the diagnosis. Sometimes, particularly in older children, only soft-tissue injuries are present. Look for bruises, burns, and bites. Intra-abdominal soft-tissue injuries are important and are now demonstrable. CT can show evidence of bowel, liver, and pancreatic injuries from blunt trauma.
- Intracranial injuries occur and are usually a result of shaking. The pathology includes: subdural haematoma, intraventricular haemorrhage, subarachnoid haemorrhage, cerebral oedema, cerebral contusion, cerebral atrophy, and hydrocephalus (Chapman and Nakielny 1995). CT and MR imaging will provide useful information.
- Your aim is not so much to diagnose child abuse as to detect possible cases and refer them to the appropriate specialist.

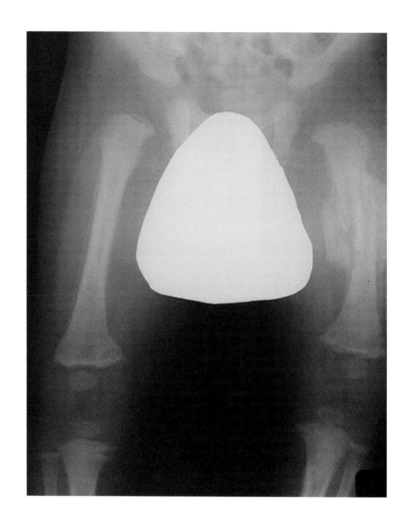

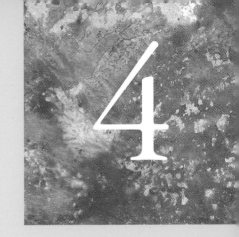

4

# Skeletal radiology: non-trauma

## Main focus and objectives

- Bone tumours:
  *How to detect the lesion*
  *How to describe it*
  *The features of benign and malignant lesions*
  *Which other modalities are available?*

- Arthritis:
  *Major criteria*
  *Minor criteria*
  *Which one and to what extent?*

- Some miscellaneous bone disorders

# Skeletal radiology: non-trauma

## Main focus and objectives

The previous chapter has covered the skills of interpreting skeletal X-rays. This chapter extends those skills to conditions other than trauma. Two important bone conditions requiring discussion are bone tumours and arthritis. In a book of this size, other diseases can only be mentioned in the captions.

Once the abnormality is detected, by knowing where to look and what to look for, proceed to interpret the abnormalities by:

- recognizing the abnormality;
- describing it in generic terms;
- giving a specific diagnosis; or
- knowing where to go to acquire that information.

The features of several common or important diseases are described below.

## Bone tumours

Bone tumours can be benign or malignant, and if malignant can be primary or secondary. They are uncommon except for secondary deposits in patients with known metastatic disease, particularly of the breast, prostate, and lung. People with the multifocal malignant disease of myeloma often have bone deposits. The other multifocal malignant diseases of leukaemia and lymphoma less commonly have bone changes.

Diagnosis of the type of tumour is a task for the specialist, but the non-specialist needs to know four things:

1. How to detect the lesion.

2. How to describe it.

3. The features of benign and malignant lesions.

4. Which other modalities are available to characterize the lesion and find the extent of the disease.

## How to detect the lesion

### Where to look

1. Look at the bone:
   - start in the centre of the bone and work outwards;
   - check the medullary cavity and trabecular pattern;
   - examine the cortex.
2. Look around the outline of the cortex for a loss of continuity or periosteal reaction.

3. Look at the joints.

4. Look at the soft tissues for any mass or swelling.

## What to look for

### Opacity:

- prostate secondaries in the male, and occasionally breast carcinoma secondaries in females, excite an osteoblastic reaction and are sclerotic
- osteosarcoma

### Radiolucency:

- most bone tumours, both benign and malignant, are radiolucent because they destroy bone

### Distortion or displacement:

- Look for expansion or collapse of a bone.
- Look for a periosteal reaction (elevation of the periosteum by pus, blood, tumour, and new bone formed on its deep surface).

## How to describe it

Start with the site, size, and shape and then describe the features from inside out:

1. Look at the matrix (footnote 10) (is it radiolucent or calcified?).

2. Look at the border, is it:
   - well defined, i.e. circumscribed or geographic (meaning like a map)—can be with or without a sclerotic margin? or
   - poorly defined?

3. Check for a periosteal reaction.

4. Look for a soft-tissue mass.

## The features of benign and malignant lesions

These are better described as indolent or aggressive lesions because this will include non-neoplastic pathology.

1. Indolent lesions (benign tumours and cysts) have features of:
   - organized new bone or calcification in the matrix (not with cysts);
   - a well-defined margin, perhaps with a thin sclerotic line;
   - an adjacent bone cortex that may be thinned or expanded;
   - no extension into the soft tissues or across the epiphyseal plate.

2. Characteristics of aggressive lesions (both aggressive benign tumours and malignant lesions, and osteomyelitis) are:
   - bone destruction;

---

10.    The intercellular substance of the bone, made up of the osteocollagenous fibres embedded in an amorphous ground substance and inorganic salts.

- irregular new bone formation;
- poorly defined margins;
- periosteal reaction or elevation;
- soft-tissue extension;
- no spread through the epiphyseal plate by tumours (but can occur with osteomyelitis).

Malignant tumours are:

- locally invasive;
- fast growing;
- metastatic;

and these features will be reflected in their appearance.

## Which other modalities are available to characterize the lesion and find the extent of the disease?

- CXR to see metastases;
- MRI to give a better image of the extent of the disease in the medullary cavity and soft tissues;
- CT scanning of the tumour site for its extent, and CT scanning of the chest to detect small pulmonary nodules;
- RNS (radionuclear scanning) to detect the tumour before it becomes visible on plain films and also to detect other bone deposits.

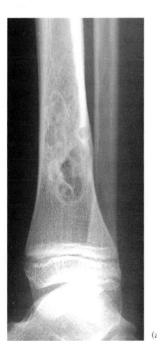

(a)

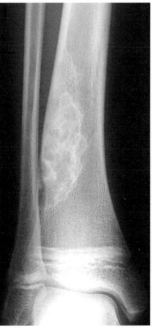

(b)

**Figs 4.1** (a), (b)  This lesion has a typical appearance and location. After you have seen a few of them it is quite acceptable to say immediately what it is. For beginners the safe way is to describe it. *Bones*: A radiolucent lesion, eccentrically placed, alignment along the long axis of the bone, involving both the cortex and medulla in the lower shaft of the tibia, the cortex being thinned and scalloped; it appears multilocular and has a sclerotic border; there is no periosteal reaction. It is an indolent lesion and the lack of fusion of the epiphysis says that it is in the bone of an adolescent. *Joints*: normal *Soft tissues*: nothing seen here The description is of a non-ossifying fibroma, a benign, localized disorder of bone growth and mineralization.

**Figs** 4.2 (a), (b)  *Bones*: The distal femur in this 19-year-old male has a poorly defined mass that has a sclerotic matrix. This is an aggressive lesion that is forming bone, hence the sclerosis. *Joint*: The patella is displaced anteriorly, signifying joint involvement. *Soft tissues*: The process has invaded the adjacent soft tissues and is generating bone formation. The likely diagnosis is an osteosarcoma. Next step is an MRI to define the extent of the tumour in the medullary cavity and in the soft tissues. The presence of lung secondaries will alter the management. A search for these can be with a CXR, but a more sensitive test is a CT scan. (more sensitive = more people with the disease will have a positive test).

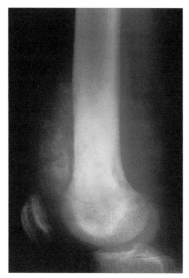
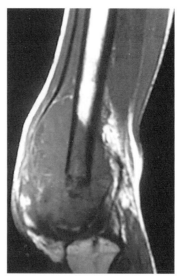

(a)                                     (b)

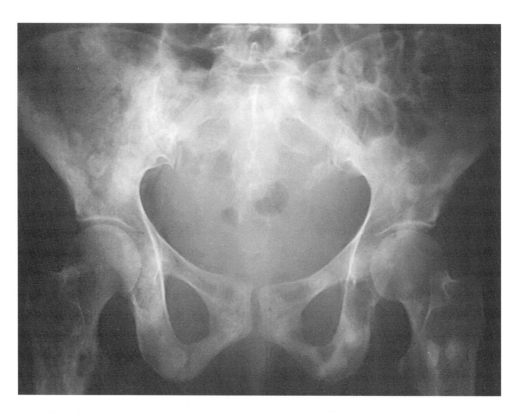

**Fig. 4.3**  *Bones*: Some of these bone lesions are lytic and some are sclerotic. They are poorly defined and one has caused destruction of the cortex of the superior margin of the right pubic bone. Carcinoma of the breast gives these mixed, lytic and sclerotic, secondaries. *Joints*: Seem to be unaffected. *Soft tissues*: normal. Most of these deposits will be asymptomatic. Pain occurs when the periosteum is involved or a pathological fracture occurs.

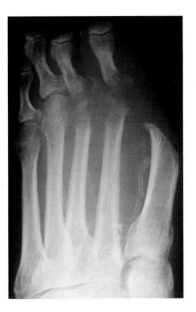

**Fig. 4.4** *Bones*: Consider the appearance of the bones around the 2nd and 3rd metatarsophalangeal joints. The abnormal radiolucency with poorly defined margins announces bone destruction. *Joints*: The distortion of joint anatomy also points to an aggressive lesion that must be either infection or tumour. Tumours do not usually spread from joint to joint. Infection can. *Soft tissues*: The foot is a common place for penetrating foreign bodies that can lead to infection. But another cause is at work here. The arterial walls are calcified, a known occurrence with diabetes mellitus. The first toe has been removed because of ischaemia or infection. This must be a case of osteomyelitis and septic arthritis, a complication of diabetes.

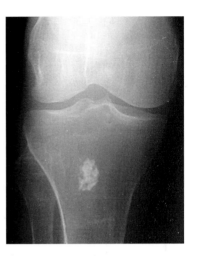

**Fig. 4.5** *Bones*: The abnormal opacity in the medullary cavity of the tibia is a well-defined, indolent lesion. It shows no evidence of aggression. This is a bone infarct. It is associated with the group of diseases that cause that other disorder of bone perfusion, avascular necrosis. *Joints*: normal *Soft tissues*: normal.

**Fig. 4.6** *Bones*: Well-defined opacities are sometimes seen in the bones and have the shape of small nodules. They are bone islands. Usually they are incidental findings and can be ignored. The problem comes when they are seen in a man of 70 years of age. Does one start a search for carcinoma of the prostate? *Joint*: normal *Soft tissues*: normal.

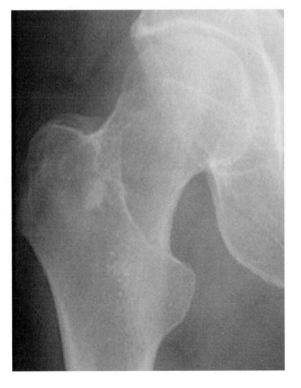

Arthritis (see footnote 11)

Non-rheumatologists do not have to know much about arthritis. However, there are some basic ideas that all doctors should understand. Try asking a friend to give you a simple definition of rheumatoid arthritis and you will realize that some people are struggling. It is difficult to diagnose and treat a disease if you don't know what it is. The definition should go something like: A chronic, systemic, inflammatory disorder probably of autoimmune aetiology, which is characterized by a proliferation of synovium (pannus formation) and consequent joint destruction, but it also involves the muscles, heart, lung, blood vessels, and skin.

Someone comes to see you. After the history is taken, the provisional diagnosis is rheumatoid arthritis. Examination and a blood test confirm the diagnosis. You order an X-ray of the hands to document the presence, extent (joints involved), and activity of the disease. What will be seen? The radiograph will reflect the pathological definition. There may be widening of the joint space because of an effusion or proliferation of pannus, or the joint space could be narrowed because of the destruction of articular cartilage, a later sign. The inflamed synovium creates a soft-tissue mass, destroys the capsule and ligaments leading to subluxation, and can attack the bone, giving erosions. Pain, lack of movement, and hyperaemia cause adjacent osteoporosis.

Some of these signs may be early changes and quite subtle. What you first need to know when looking at the film is, *Are there changes which confirm the presence of arthritis?* Answer yes if there is one *major* criterion or a *minor* criterion with additional evidence of arthritis, such as a second minor criterion.

## Major criteria for diagnosing current or past arthritis on X-rays

Only one of the following needed:

- joint space narrowing;

- osteophyte formation or subchondral sclerosis;

- periarticular bone erosion.

## Minor criteria

Supporting evidence is needed because these signs occur with other disease processes:

- joint space widening from an effusion, pus or pannus (can also occur with haemarthrosis);

- chondrocalcinosis (footnote 12) (can occur in elderly people with no other indication of active arthritis);

---

11.  Arthritis = inflammation of a joint, but by common usage includes non-inflammatory conditions such as osteoarthrosis.

- arthritides = plural of arthritis

- arthropathy = something wrong with the joint

12.  Calcification of the articular cartilage or menisci.

- juxta-articular demineralization (but it can also occur with disuse osteoporosis and Sudeck's atrophy);

- alignment abnormalities, subluxation (can also occur with trauma);

- diffusely swollen digit; indicates psoriatic arthritis (can also occur with infection);

- soft-tissue swelling (can also occur with trauma and soft-tissue infection).

## Which one and to what extent?

Once it is clear that arthritis is present the questions are, 'Which one?' and 'To what extent?' Radiographs will reveal the joints involved and help answer both these questions. Comparison with previous films will give an indication of activity.

If only one joint is involved (monoarticular), there is no trick:

Osteoarthrosis

Trauma

Rheumatoid arthritis

Infection

Crystal-induced arthropathy (gout and pseudogout).

If the disease is polyarticular, the answer is usually one of four groups (from the International Classification of Diseases, ICD):

- diffuse connective tissue disease, such as rheumatoid arthritis;

- arthritis associated with spondylitis (i.e. spondyloarthritis) formerly called seronegative rheumatoid variants—seronegative means negative for rheumatoid factor, spondylitis is inflammatory arthritis of the spine;

- osteoarthrosis;

- metabolic and endocrine diseases associated with rheumatic states.

The most common diffuse connective tissue disease is rheumatoid arthritis. It has a swollen, inflamed synovium that erodes the bone, and destroys cartilage, joint capsules, and ligaments. The X-ray will show these changes. This type of arthritis is distinguished by periarticular erosions, joint-space narrowing, alignment abnormalities, and juxta-articular demineralization (periarticular osteoporosis from a lack of movement and increased perfusion of the bone ends because of the inflammation). In 80% of cases, rheumatoid arthritis is seropositive. The other types of the diffuse connective tissue diseases include juvenile arthritis, lupus erythematosis, and forms of necrotizing vasculitis which produce arthritis.

The spondyloarthritides are a group of inflammatory diseases that have a predilection for the spine and the sacroiliac joints and for asymmetrical involvement of the peripheral joints. They are: ankylosing spondylitis, psoriatic arthritis, enteropathic arthritis, and Reiter's disease.

Osteoarthrosis (OA) is also called osteoarthritis, and degenerative joint disease (DJD). It is characterized radiologically by osteophytes and uneven joint-space narrowing. Usually a primary disorder, it involves, as you know, the hips, knees, distal interphalangeal joints, and spine. It can also develop secondary to any other disease that attacks and weakens the joints, such as rheumatoid arthritis, gout, congenital hip dislocation, or trauma.

*Hint*

Seriously consider aspirating the joint in cases of monoarticular arthritis to make the diagnosis. Septic arthritis must not be missed. Infectious arthritis can be pyogenic, granulomatous (TB), fungal or viral.

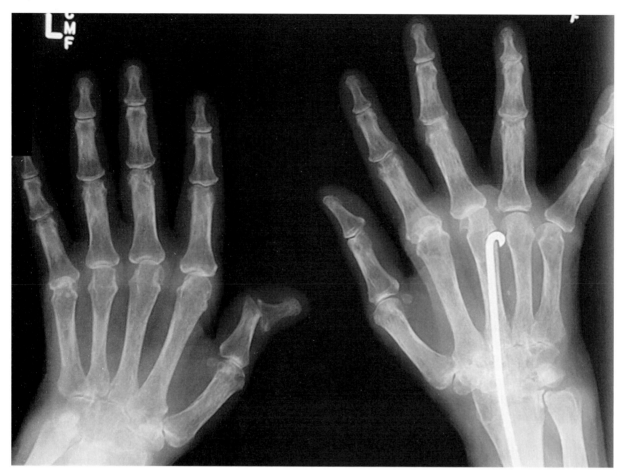

**Fig. 4.7** *Bones*: Osteoporotic with erosions of heads of the metacarpals and proximal phalanges. Destruction of the carpal bones of the right wrist. *Joints*: Narrowing of the joint spaces, and subluxation of the interphalangeal joint of the left thumb and of several of the metacarpophalangeal joints. *Soft tissues*: swelling. Arthritis is present because two of the major criteria are present: joint space narrowing and erosions. Two minor criteria are also fulfilled: subluxation and juxta-articular osteoporosis. Now to decide which type. It is polyarticular, so infection is out. This is an example of an arthritis which is relatively symmetrical, has destroyed articular cartilage, attacked the capsule and ligaments leading to alignment abnormalities, eroded the bone particularly where it is not covered by cartilage, destroyed the right wrist carpal joints requiring internal fixation, caused soft-tissue swelling, and led to osteoporosis secondary to pain, immobility, and hyperaemia. It is an inflammatory disorder, rheumatoid arthritis.

Metabolic and endocrine diseases are suspected of causing arthritis when there are soft-tissue masses, periarticular erosions, and chondrocalcinosis but with a normal width of joint space. The most common are the crystal-associated conditions, i.e. the crystal deposition diseases of gout and pseudogout. They induce an inflammatory reaction both within and outside the joint. Many other biochemical abnormalities such as inborn errors of metabolism and endocrine diseases can cause arthritis.

This is about the limit of complexity in describing arthritis that should be achieved in this book. It forms a framework onto which other knowledge can be added when needed, and if needed, by association—a mental hook.

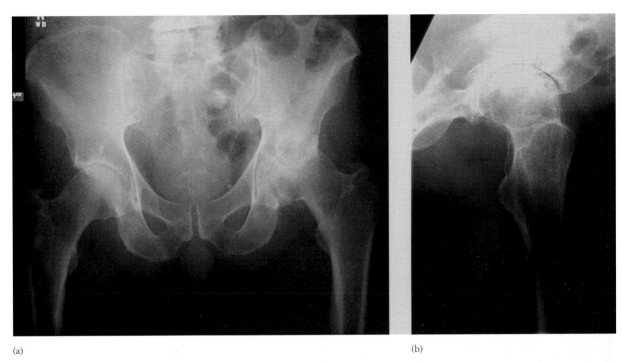

(a)                                                                                      (b)

**Figs 4.8** (a) and (b)  *Bones*: Subarticular sclerosis and cystic changes of the left acetabulum and head of the femur. The head of the femur is distorted (flattened). *Joints*: The joint space of the left hip is narrowed. These are the changes of osteoarthrosis.

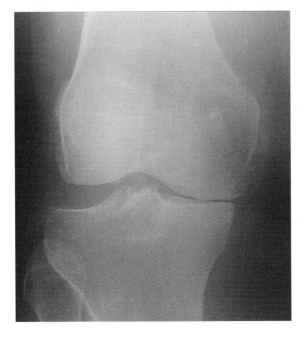

**Fig. 4.9**  A weight-bearing radiograph. *Bones*: The subarticular bone is becoming sclerotic but the osteophytes have not yet developed. *Joint*: Is there arthritis in this joint? Definitely. One of the major criteria of arthritis, joint-space narrowing, is present, signalling loss of articular cartilage. The tibia is subluxed laterally on the femur. This is osteoarthrosis. Why is the medial compartment affected while the lateral is spared? That is one of the mysteries of life. Current thinking is that the cause may be a metabolic disturbance of the articular cartilage.

**Fig.** 4.10 *Bones*: Osteophytes are developing, shown by sharpening of the corners of the femur and tibia. *Joint*: Abnormal opacification of the fibrocartilage has affected the menisci. It is called chondrocalcinosis. Chondrocalcinosis can also affect the articular cartilage. It occurs in calcium pyrophosphate dihydrate deposition disease (CPPD), osteoarthrosis, gout, haemochromatosis, and Wilson's disease. The diagnosis of chondrocalcinosis is made on the X-ray. The diagnosis of the type of arthritis often requires aspiration and examination of the joint fluid. Calcium pyrophosphate arthropathy is *chronic* CPPD deposition disease with radiographic changes of chondrocalcinosis, joint-space narrowing, subchondral sclerosis, and osteophytes. Pseudogout is *acute* CPPD deposition disease with pain like an attack of acute gout but often with no radiological changes. Often acute gout also has no radiological changes except perhaps soft-tissue swelling

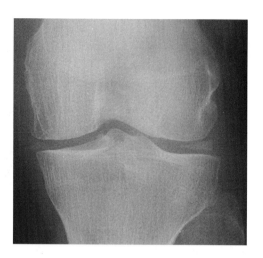

## Some miscellaneous bone disorders

**Fig.** 4.11 *Bones*: An obvious deformity of the medial femoral condyle. *Joint*: A bone fragment lies nearby. This disease process affects articular surfaces which are convex and is probably related to loss of blood supply and chronic injury, although the exact cause is unknown. It also can affect the head of the humerus and the convex articular surface of the talus. It is osteochondritis dissecans.

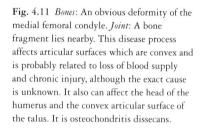

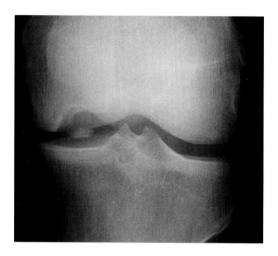

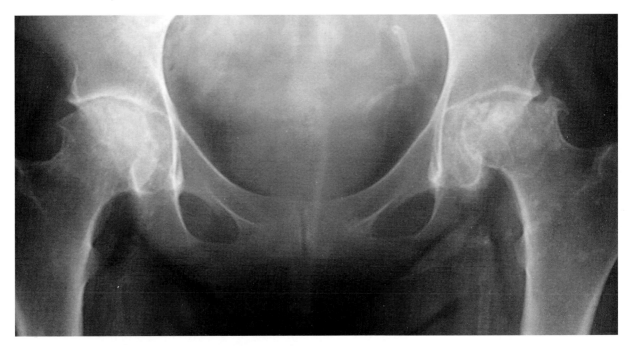

**Fig. 4.12** *Bones*: The femoral heads seem sclerotic and their shape is distorted, particularly that on the left which is destroyed superiorly on the weight-bearing cortex. *Joints*: The loss of articular cartilage in the hips is noticeable, but strangely, the acetabular bone is little affected. The disease is therefore one of the head of the femur rather than an arthropathy. It is avascular necrosis. Another joint is the symphysis pubis. It has narrowing and irregularity of the articular surfaces, seen in osteitis pubis, a common degenerative or inflammatory disorder. *Soft tissues*: The search is continued for any other opacity, radiolucency, or distortion or displacement and another finding is returned, calcification of the walls of the muscular arteries. This occurs with atherosclerosis and is more pronounced with diabetes.

**Fig. 4.13** *Bones*: Something is wrong with the right femur. It is a diffuse process that causes coarsening of the trabecular pattern, thickened cortex, and bone sclerosis. Additionally, there are fractures, called incremental fractures, of the lateral cortex. These result from tensile (distracting) forces, compared with the compressive forces affecting the medial cortex. The femur is becoming bowed because the bone quality is poor. This must be Paget's disease in the late phase of sclerosis. The disease is one of abnormal bone metabolism and passes through two earlier stages, one being osteolytic and the other mixed osteolytic–osteoblastic. *Joints*: The hip joint has the loss of cartilage that occurs with osteoarthrosis. *Soft tissues*: The atherosclerotic vessels have calcified plaque, allowing demonstration of the bifurcation of the common femoral artery into the superficial femoral artery and the profunda femoris artery. Correlate this with the diagram of the blood supply to the head of the femur following fractures of the femoral neck.

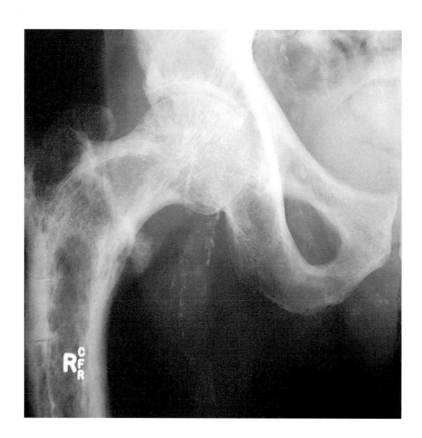

**Figs 4.14** (a), (b)  A history of trauma. *Bones*: There is no evidence of a fracture line. The two white lines in the lower tibia could be from a compression fracture but the cortex is intact. The proximal line is a growth line or growth-arrest line caused by some temporary metabolic disturbance in the past. It is classed as a normal variant. The distal line is the remnant of the epiphyseal plate as the epiphysis fuses with the metaphysis. *Joints*: In cases of trauma always look for subluxation. Make sure there is no abnormal widening of the distal tibiofibular joint (a syndesmosis). Difficult to judge, however, as the normal width varies considerably

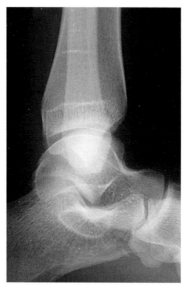

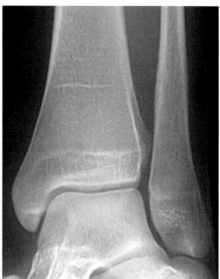

(a)　　　　　　　　　　　　　(b)

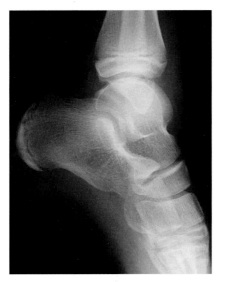

(a)

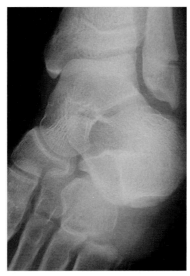

(b)

**Figs** 4.15 (a), (b) *Bones*: the radiolucency near the end of the bone is where bone growth is proceeding. It is called the growth plate or physis or epiphyseal plate, but not the 'epiphysis'. That name is reserved for the bone between the epiphyseal plate and the articular surface. The epiphyseal plate is radiolucent because, like the articular cartilage, it is not calcified. Scanning these films reveals two apparent abnormalities, an opaque epiphysis of the calcaneus and an apophysis (footnote 13) of the base of the 5th metatarsal, both normal appearances. An avulsion fracture of the base of the metatarsal, because of the tug of the peroneus brevis, would have a transverse fracture line. *Joints*: normal.

---

13.  Like an epiphysis but it does not add to the length of the bone.

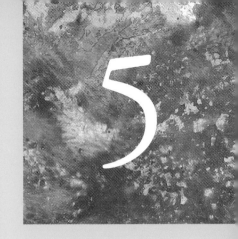

# 5

# Acute radiology of the head and spine

## Main focus and objectives

- Trauma to the head:
  *CT of the head*
  *Skull X-rays*
  *Facial bones*

- Trauma to the cervical spine:
  *Lateral cervical spine view*
  *The AP peg view*
  *The AP film*
  *What happens next?*

- How to look at the thoracic spine

- How to look at the lumbar spine

- Some diseases of the spine:

# Acute radiology of the head and spine

## Main focus and objectives

This chapter examines trauma to the head, trauma to the cervical spine, and non-traumatic diseases of the head and spine.

The objective is to give a system of interpretation of head and spine X-rays, and CT of the head, focusing on:

(1) normal radiological anatomy;

(2) how to look at images of plain films and CT:

    (a) where to look:

        (i) following a logical perceptual flow

        (ii) important sites

    (b) what to look for:

        (i) abnormal opacity

        (ii) abnormal radiolucency

        (iii) distortion or displacement of a normal structure;

(3) how to interpret the abnormalities by:

    (a) recognizing the abnormality,

    (b) describing it in generic terms,

    (c) giving a specific diagnosis, or

    (d) knowing where to go to get that information;

(4) features of several diseases, trauma and non-trauma.

## Trauma to the head

Trauma to the head can be penetrating or non-penetrating.

Penetrating injuries occur from bullets and sharp instruments. Imaging is directed to revealing where they went and what damage was done on the way. CT is the most useful modality. Metal and magnets (MRI) do not mix. Pay careful attention to a patient with a history of hammering metal on metal and feeling something hit the eye. Plain films or a CT are necessary to exclude an intraocular foreign body.

Acceleration–deceleration or rotational forces cause blunt or non-penetrating trauma. These forces damage the skull, intracranial contents, face, and cervical spine. They are associated with injuries elsewhere in the body and can cause difficulties in deciding what to treat first.

Skull fractures are not a problem, except if they tear a meningeal artery or are depressed or expand as a child grows.

Within hours, a severed meningeal artery produces an extradural haematoma that strips the dura off the inner table of the skull. The haematoma cannot extend beyond where the dura is firmly attached, such as at the coronal and sagittal sutures. The CT appearance is often of a biconvex or lentiform (lens-shaped), high attenuation mass separating the cerebral hemisphere from the skull. Blood is of high attenuation because of the protein concentration. There will be mass effect. The brain will be compressed as will the lateral ventricle on that side. Herniation can occur; across to the contralateral side (subfalcine herniation) and into the posterior fossa (uncal herniation) through the tentorial hiatus.

Subdural haematomas form more slowly, often over days, and sometimes in a stop–start manner. The bleeding comes from bridging veins which cross from the cerebral cortex to the skull. These veins are stretched in people who have some loss of brain substance perhaps secondary to atherosclerosis or ageing. The veins are torn when a rotational force is applied to the skull. The blood fills and expands the space between the dura and the arachnoid and therefore can extend past the coronal suture. The falx cerebri will contain it to one side of the cranial cavity.

Imaging of trauma to the head is essentially with CT, X-rays of the facial bones, orthopantomograms (OPG), and occasionally skull X-rays.

## CT of the head

Who needs a CT of the head following trauma? The easy decision is to order a CT for everyone, but that causes expense, less availability of the scanner for those who really need it, and radiation to the head—particularly the lens of the eye. Various guidelines have been introduced. They suggest a CT for someone with significant trauma, loss of consciousness, amnesia, or neurological symptoms or signs. Check the local rules.

## How to look at a CT of the head

### Where to look

1. Check the ventricles: lateral; third; fourth.

## What to look for

### Distortion:

- *Site*: shift of the ventricles is usually caused by a space-occupying lesion (SOL) such as a haematoma, tumour, or oedema; uncommonly by negative mass effect of an old infarct.
- *Size*: small with an SOL or overshunting; large = ventriculomegaly and occurs with communicating or non-communicating hydrocephalus, and cerebral atrophy.
- *Shape*: compressed by a mass or oedema; the Arnold–Chiari malformation gives the ventricles a strange shape.

2. Check the cerebral and cerebellar attenuation.

## What to look for

### Opacity: increased attenuation

- In the precontrast scan, calcification is often seen in the pineal gland, choroid plexus, and basal ganglia in older patients. Increased attenuation also occurs with haemorrhage and some tumours: meningioma, melanoma; and colonic adenocarcinoma secondaries.
- In the postcontrast scan, increased attenuation is seen with any lesion where there is abundant perfusion or breakdown of the blood–brain barrier. Normally, in the body, intravenous contrast is distributed throughout the intravascular and extravascular components of the extracellular space, except in the brain where the blood–brain barrier excludes it. The breakdown of this barrier occurs with tumours because of their abnormal capillary development and with inflammatory lesions with their loose endothelial junctions. Cerebral infarcts sometimes show contrast enhancement in the infarcted tissue and also in the ischaemic tissue surrounding the infarct after several days. This results from perfusion being re-established and the formation of new capillaries, but no effective blood–brain barrier.

### Radiolucency: decreased attenuation with oedema

- Cytotoxic oedema, as the name implies, appears with cell death from infarction and has a distribution consistent with the blood supply.
- Vasogenic oedema spreads through the white matter and is caused by tumours or inflammation. The tumours themselves, whether primary or secondary, are often less dense than normal brain tissue on the precontrast scan.
- Periventricular oedema is seen around the anterior and posterior horns of the lateral ventricles in atherosclerotic encephalopathy and non-communicating hydrocephalus.
- Herpes encephalitis is low attenuation but often has areas of haemorrhage.

### Distortion:

- Distortion of the grey and white matter of the cerebrum and cerebellum occurs with any space-occupying lesion: a tumour, haemorrhage, oedema, or inflammatory mass.

3. Check the skull, orbits, and facial structures.

## What to look for

### Opacity:

- fluid in the paranasal sinuses, indirect evidence of a fracture

### Radiolucency:

- fracture of the skull or facial bones
- gas in the soft tissues.

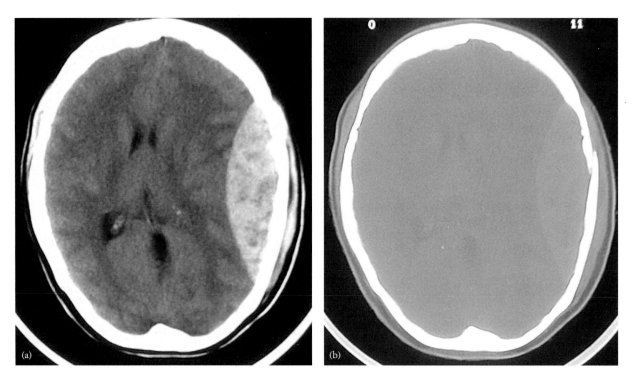

**Figs 5.1** (a), (b) *Ventricles*: These are distorted, compressed, and shifted to the right. Only the calcified choroid plexus remains to be seen of the posterior horn of the left lateral ventricle. *Cerebral hemispheres*: The left hemisphere is compressed and shifted across with subfalcine herniation. On another, lower, slice one would look for uncal herniation. A good descriptor for the high-density shape, superficial to the left cerebral hemisphere, is fusiform (spindle-shaped), lentiform (lens-shaped), or biconvex. It is limited anteriorly by the coronal suture and posteriorly by the lambdoid suture, these being strong attachments of the dura to the skull. This is an extradural haematoma and to strip the dura from the inner table of the skull requires high pressure (arterial). *Bones*: The fracture that has torn a branch of the middle meningeal artery is shown with the window and level (footnote 14) manipulated to demonstrate the bones.

14. Many CT scanners calculate the attenuation (how much of the X-ray beam is absorbed or deflected) of tissue as a scale of $-1000$ (air) to $+3000$. The units are called Hounsfield units (HU) or CT numbers. If a window width of 80, centred at a level of 40, is chosen for display, anything that has the attenuation of water (0 HU) or less will appear black. Brain tissue will be grey. Blood (80 HU) and anything with more attenuation will be white. Widening the window will *decrease* the contrast.

The *level* is where the window is centred. Selecting a higher level will make the image appear darker. At quite high levels only the bones will be seen, everything else will look black. The terms 'window' and 'level' are not the same as 'contrast' and 'brightness'.

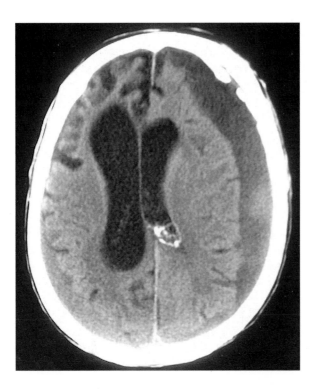

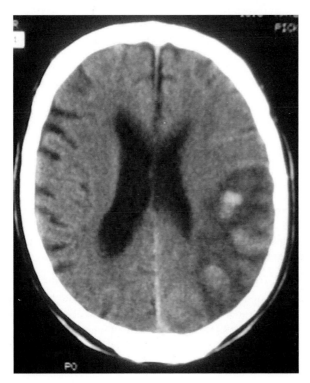

**Fig. 5.2 *Ventricles*:** The lateral ventricles are shifted to the right and are enlarged, particularly the right. *Cerebral hemispheres*: The left cerebral hemisphere is compressed, has small sulci, and is in turn compressing and displacing the lateral ventricle under the falx–subfalcine herniation. The cause of the problem is a crescent-shaped radiolucency between the left cerebral cortex and the skull. It was blood but the haemoglobin has been reabsorbed, leaving serum. A poorly defined area of increased attenuation in the fluid indicates a recent bleed. The pathogenesis of this subdural haematoma is clear from this image. The cerebral hemispheres are small and atrophic. The bridging veins from the cortex to the skull are stretched and easily torn by minor trauma such as quickly turning the head (rotational injury). It is always wise to look systematically at the film after being distracted by the obvious abnormality. Check the ventricles (site, size, and configuration), the cerebral and cerebellar attenuation, and the *skull and facial bones*. Part of the choroid plexus is calcified. A smaller subdural haematoma is on the right side posteriorly. It is more recent as it is more dense than the other, isodense with the brain.

**Fig. 5.3** One image of a plain (without IV contrast) CT head scan. This 84-year-old man had a CVA (cerebrovascular accident) 5 days earlier and fell out of bed. CT scan to exclude an extradural or subdural haematoma. *Ventricles*: The left lateral ventricle is distorted/compressed. *Cerebral hemispheres*: a circumscribed area of low attenuation in the left parietal lobe. Low attenuation usually means fluid. In this case it is oedema, from an infarct of part of the territory of the middle cerebral artery. It has caused mass effect with compression of the left lateral ventricle and the cerebral sulci on that side. Over the last 5 days the thrombolytic factors in the blood have caused the clot, be it a thrombus or embolus, to break up. The fragments have moved distally, allowing perfusion of ischaemic tissue with damaged vessel walls. These walls have given way under the systolic pressure and haemorrhage has occurred into the infarct, with the abnormal opacity being blood. The diagnosis is a haemorrhagic infarct. Understanding pathology makes the images easy, or at least not as difficult.

## Skull X-rays

Skull X-rays for trauma should only be performed when CT or MRI are unavailable, although some would recommend their use in cases of a suspected depressed fracture, penetrating injury, or in children under 2 years of age with a head injury, to detect non-accidental injury (Lloyd *et al.* 1997).

### How to look at skull X-rays

- Check the name.
- Is there any rotation?

Where to look

- Check centrally and then around the margins.

# What to look for

### Opacity:

- Linear or curvilinear density of superimposed bone indicates a depressed fracture.
- Fluid in the sphenoid sinus suggests a fracture of the base of the skull.

### Radiolucency:

- A fracture line is straighter, has sharper margins, and is in different sites than vascular channels and sutures.
- Pneumocephalus: gas is present in the anterior cranial fossa in a supine patient.

### Displacement of a normal structure:

- A calcified pineal gland may be shifted from the midline when seen in the frontal projection. This is an old sign of an extradural or subdural haematoma.

## Facial bones

The facial bones appear complicated because of the superimposition of structures. Looking at three features—the orbits, the maxillary sinuses, and the zygomatic arches—in the frontal projection will detect most fractures.

1. The orbits. Check the margins, adjacent frontal and ethmoidal sinuses, and the orbital contents.
2. The maxillary sinuses. Look at the margins and the contents.

   Facial bone radiographs are best taken with a horizontal beam, which means that if fluid is present in a sinus a fluid level will be visible. This is indirect evidence of a fracture. Sometimes the fracture itself cannot be seen.
3. The zygomatic arches. The arch has the appearance of an elephant's head and trunk (Dolan *et al.* 1978).

# What to look for (orbits)

*Opacity:*

- Fluid in the sinuses

*Radiolucency:*

- Look for a fracture line.
- Gas can sometimes be seen in the orbit as a crescent-shaped radiolucency above the globe, indicating a fracture involving the ethmoid or maxillary sinus.

*Distortion:*

- A fracture, if displaced, will cause irregularity of the orbital margin. A blow-out fracture causes prolapse of the orbital contents into the ethmoid or maxillary sinuses.

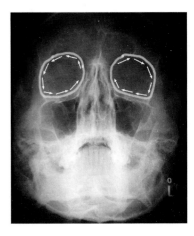

Fig. 5.4 Looking at the orbits.

# What to look for (maxillary sinuses)

*Opacity:*

- fluid in the sinus
- soft tissue protruding from the orbit

*Radiolucency:*

- fracture line

*Distortion:*

- loss of continuity of the bony margin

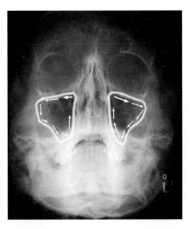

Fig. 5.5 Looking at the maxillary sinuses.

Views of the mandible need to be requested specifically as they are not included in the facial bone series. An OPG (orthopantomogram) sometimes shows the fracture and position of the fragments more clearly than AP and oblique views.

# What to look for (zygomatic arches)

*Radiolucency:*

- fracture

*Distortion:*

- depressed fracture of the arch

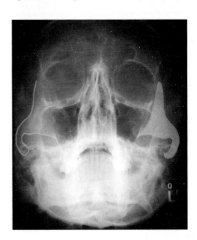

Fig. 5.6 Looking at the zygomatic arches.

**Fig. 5.7** This film is taken PA, that is with the facial bones next to the film cassette, in order to have a sharper image and less magnification of the important structures. Because much of the beam is attenuated by the head, the lens of the eye receives less radiation than it would have with an AP film, an important consideration as it is a radiosensitive structure. The facial bones seem like a busy film but there are only three areas to cover to detect most abnormalities:

(1) *orbits*: fractures of the lateral and inferior margins of the left orbit;

(2) *maxillary sinuses*: fracture of the lateral wall of the left maxillary sinus with a haematoma lifting the mucoperiosteum to give an opacity;

(3) *zygomatic arches*: fracture of the left zygoma

This is called a tripod fracture as the zygoma is separated at its three attachments to the other facial bones, often from a fist or some other blunt object.

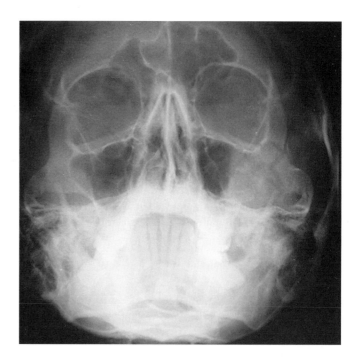

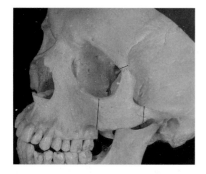

**Fig. 5.8** Tripod fracture of the facial bones.

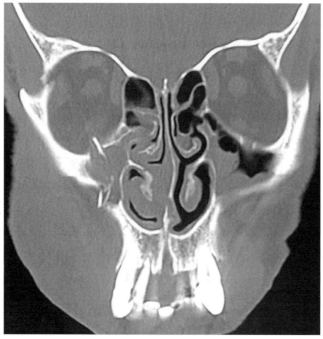

**Fig. 5.9** CT images are difficult to teach in a book because only one or two images can be presented and much of the interpretation depends on comparing the image with the slices above and below. Two of the fractures of a tripod fracture are visible: lateral wall of the right orbit and the walls of the maxillary sinus. The third will be in the zygomatic arch. Polypoid swelling of the mucoperiosteum in the left maxillary sinus is seen and indicates sinusitis.

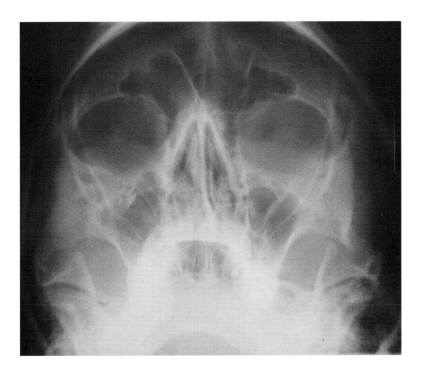

**Fig. 5.10** *Orbits*: Looking at the orbits will reveal the relative opacity caused by soft-tissue swelling over the left cheekbone (or zygoma for those in the know). *Maxillary sinus*: The outline of the left one is unremarkable. *Zygoma*: The shape of the left is distorted. The *zygomatic arch* exhibits a depressed fracture

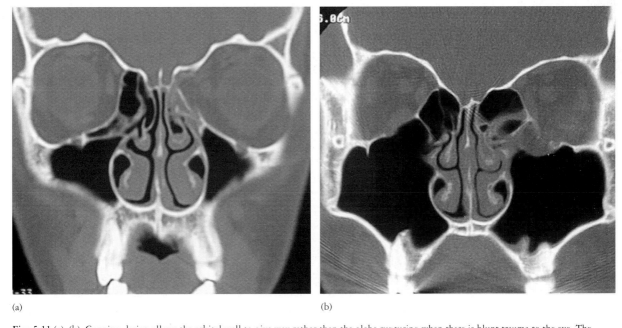

(a)                                                                                          (b)

**Figs 5.11** (a), (b) Cunning design allows the orbital wall to give way rather than the globe rupturing when there is blunt trauma to the eye. The result is a blow-out fracture, into the ethmoid sinus or into the maxillary sinus. Fat and the rectus muscle can be trapped in the sinus, causing diplopia. Figure (a) shows a blow-out fracture involving the left ethmoid sinus. In figure (b) the soft tissue protrudes into the maxillary sinus in another patient.

**Fig. 5.12** An unusual case of someone with all 32 teeth: two incisors, one canine, two premolars, and three molars, × 4. This orthopantomogram (OPG) demonstrates a fracture of the right side of the body. An oblique and a PA view can also be done, as fractures of the mandible are not always easy to see. The pull of muscles causes the displacement of the fragments. Because of the adherence of the mucous membrane to the mandible in the mouth, the fracture will tear the mucous membrane, making this an open fracture. Interestingly, these fractures rarely become infected. Look carefully at the condylar neck, angle and body of the mandible for evidence of a second fracture.

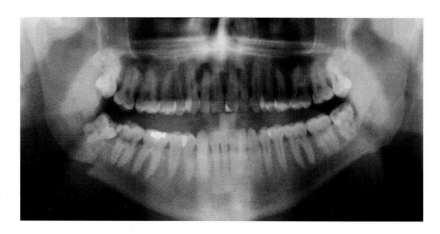

## Trauma to the cervical spine

Cervical spine radiographs should always be performed in a patient who has suffered trauma and is unconscious, and in conscious people with symptoms or signs to warrant this investigation. It requires sharp clinical skills to decide how much investigation is appropriate. A whiplash injury, for example, may need no imaging, a single lateral view, flexion and extension views, or an extensive series of plain films together with CT and MRI. It depends on the velocity of the impact, underlying diseases, symptoms, signs, and local guidelines. Remember that any imaging study is a limited examination; further views can always be ordered. There is a trade-off of the pursuit of certainty, balanced against the limit of resources.

The lateral projection contains the most information of the standard three views. The two others are the AP and the peg view.

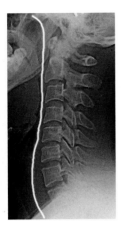

**Fig. 5.13** Perceptual flow: prevertebral tissues.

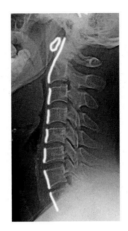

**Fig. 5.14** Perceptual flow: anterior alignment.

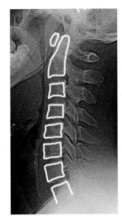

**Fig. 5.15** Perceptual flow: vertebral bodies.

## Lateral cervical spine view

### *Where to look*

The perceptual flow is up and down and from anterior to posterior.

Check that all seven vertebrae are visible, as well as the C7–T1 disc, and at least the superior part of T1. If the C7–T1 junction is not visible, obtain a swimmer's (footnote 15) view, oblique views, or a CT.

Start at the posterior borders of the rami of the mandibles. They should be aligned if there is no rotation.

Look down the prevertebral space to see if it is widened by a haematoma. A useful rule is that it should not be wider than 30% of the AP diameter of the body of C3 at that level, and at the level of C7 not more than 100% of the width of the body. A nasogastric tube *in situ* will annul this rule.

Follow the line of the anterior longitudinal ligament, looking for displacement.

Check the vertebral bodies from C1 to C7. Look carefully at the odontoid process.

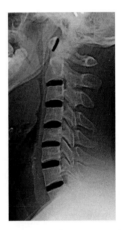

**Fig. 5.16** Perceptual flow: intervertebral discs.

Next, look at the 'black' parts. Make sure the C7–T1 disc space is shown and then examine all the spaces up to C2–C3. The atlantodens interval should be included here. It is increased when the cruciate ligament is ruptured. The width should *not* be more than 3 mm in adults or 5 mm in children.

Look down along the posterior surfaces of the vertebral bodies.

Starting from C7, check that the apophyseal joint surfaces are parallel.

The junction of the spinous processes and the laminae, called the spinolaminar line, is examined from above down. It should form a smooth curve.

Finally, check the interspinous distances for abnormal widening which occurs in hyperflexion injuries with rupture of the supraspinous and interspinous ligaments.

15. A lateral view taken with one arm up and one arm down as if swimming freestyle. It removes the superimposition of the shoulders that attenuate too many photons.

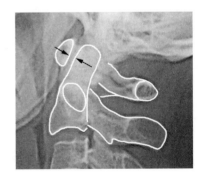

**Fig. 5.17** Atlantodens interval.

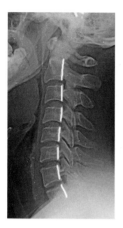

**Fig. 5.18** Perceptual flow: posterior alignment.

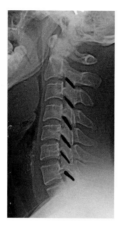

**Fig. 5.19** Perceptual flow: apophyseal joints.

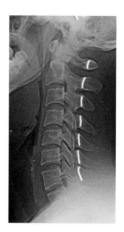

**Fig. 5.20** Perceptual flow: spinolaminar line.

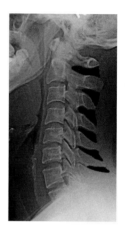

**Fig. 5.21** Perceptual flow: interspinous distances.

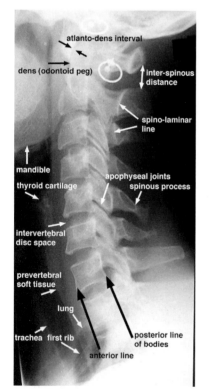

atlanto-dens interval

dens (odontoid peg)

inter-spinous distance

spino-laminar line

mandible

thyroid cartilage

apophyseal joints
spinous process

intervertebral disc space

prevertebral soft tissue

lung

trachea  first rib

posterior line of bodies

anterior line

**Fig. 5.22** Lateral C spine

## What to look for (lateral cervical spine view)

### Radiolucency:

- fracture line in the body, odontoid process, pedicle, lamina, or spinous process

### Distortion or displacement:

- Prevertebral space = haematoma.
- Malalignment of vertebrae = rupture of ligaments and subluxation/dislocation. Can have a unifacet or bifacet dislocation of the apophyseal joints.
- Crushed vertebra.
- A widened disc space indicates a serious hyperextension injury.
- A narrowed disc space suggests a crushed disc. A fragment can project posteriorly. An MRI may be required.
- Hyperflexion injuries may rupture the interspinous and supraspinous ligaments giving a widened interspinous distance.
- With a severe hyperextension injury the vertebral bodies are sometimes torn apart but then come together again and look as though nothing has happened.

## The AP peg view

### Where to look

- Look at the occipital condyles, lateral masses of C1, and the odontoid peg, body, and lateral masses of C2.
- Check the joint spaces of the atlanto-occipital and atlantoaxial joints.

## What to look for

### Opacity:

- Overlapping or compressed bone fragments

### Radiolucency:

- fracture

### Distortion or displacement:

- Look for loss of alignment of the atlanto-occipital and C1–C2 apophyseal joints.
- Look for the dens not lying midway between the lateral masses of C1, caused by a C1–C2 subluxation, or rotation of the head or neck.
- Look for an irregularity of the bony cortex.

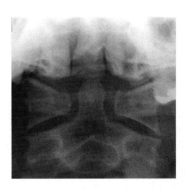

**Fig. 5.23** Normal peg view.

## The AP film

### Where to look

Start at the middle and work outwards. Look at the white parts (bones) first. Check:

- the alignment of the spinous processes and their distance from each other—the spinous processes are often bifid;
- the vertebral bodies;
- pedicles;
- lateral masses.

Look also at the upper thoracic spine and the first ribs and medial ends of the clavicles.

Once happy with the bones, check the joint spaces, the disc spaces, and the unco-vertebral joints.

## What to look for

### Radiolucency:

- fracture of the lateral masses

### Displacement or distortion:

- loss of alignment of the spinous processes or widening of the spaces between them.
- subluxation of a vertebral body

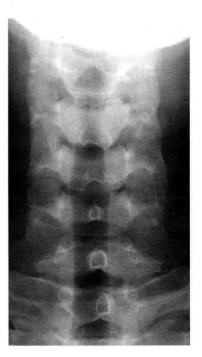

**Fig. 5.24** Normal AP cervical spine.

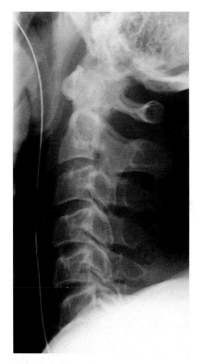

**Fig. 5.25** A nasogastric tube is in place. A collar stabilizes the neck and a circular clip is visible near the spinous process of C5. At first glance there does not appear to be much wrong, but following the system will disclose a major abnormality. Only the upper 6 cervical vertebrae are seen in this 54-year-old man. Further views are required to show T1. Following the anterior alignment of the bodies reveals a step at C5–6. The disc space at that level is widened anteriorly. Another step is seen in the alignment of the posterior cortex of the vertebral bodies. The more one looks at this level, the easier it is to see the incongruity. This is a hyperextension injury with rupture of the anterior and posterior longitudinal ligaments and intervertebral disc, together with subluxation. No sign of a haematoma anteriorly. Not every sign is present in every case.

Flexion and extension views are useful for demonstrating subluxation or stability but should only be requested by medical staff experienced in cervical trauma. It is important that the patient be asked to move his head, i.e. an active movement. Passive movement of the neck for diagnostic purposes should *not* be performed.

CT gives more information about fractures. MRI demonstrates disc disease and damage to the spinal cord such as contusion. These images may be needed if there is a fracture, subluxation, radiculopathy, or long tract signs.

## What happens next?

Many X-rays of the cervical spine appear to be normal. What happens next? Consider this scenario:

A 25-year-old female is brought to your hospital following a motor-cycle accident. A three-view cervical spine series is ordered and when it comes back, it looks both adequate and normal. Let us say that 90% of fractures and subluxations will be picked up on these three plain films. Do you stop there or continue with oblique views, flexion/extension views, C.T, or MRI?

It depends.

*On what?*

On what you thought *before* you ordered the cervical spine X-ray.

If a fracture or subluxation was unlikely, further views are probably unnecessary.

If a fracture or subluxation was likely, and yet not seen, further imaging is essential.

The decision about what to do if the test is normal needs to be made *before* the test is ordered.

*Why?*

Because in a few cases the test may miss the pathology.

The safety net is that, with the aid of the history and examination, you can allocate a pretest probability:

- Low probability means accept the negative test and treat appropriately.

- High pretest probability means: do not accept a negative result as it may be a false-negative. Return to thinking: 'What do I need to know?' and 'Which further test will provide that information?'

The pretest probability is important because it:

- determines what you will do when the X-ray comes back, whether it be positive or negative;

- provides feedback about what you thought was there and what now appears to be there, honing your clinical judgement;

- clarifies your thoughts; and

- helps you to think through what needs to be confirmed, excluded, defined, or followed up.

## How to look at the thoracic spine

It is not always easy to know exactly which vertebra is which. Sometimes it does not matter. When it does, count the vertebrae in the AP film from the top and also from the bottom to check. The last rib is sometimes small and only recognized because it angles downwards. The lumbar transverse processes project laterally. In the lateral projection, follow the last rib to find T12. There is not much joy in trying to count from above.

Devise a search pattern for yourself similar to that of the lumbar spine.

## How to look at the lumbar spine

Count how many lumbar vertebrae there are and correlate the levels in the lateral and frontal projections. The iliac crests can be seen on both views and are usually at the level of the L4–L5 disc. Check the alignment. There can be a scoliosis, convex either to the right or left, and an increase or decrease of the normal lumbar lordosis.

### Lateral view

#### Where to look

Start at the front and work backwards

(1)  prevertebral tissues

(2)  anterior alignment of the bodies

(3)  vertebral bodies and sacrum

(4)  intervertebral discs

(5)  posterior alignment of the bodies

(6)  pars interarticulares

(7)  spinous processes

## What to look for

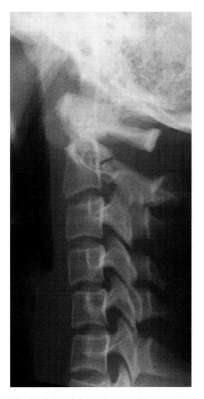

**Fig. 5.26** Many fractures and subluxations are at the C1–C2 and the C7–T1 levels. This fracture will be seen because of a radiolucency in the pedicle. The displacement of the posterior element of C2 is disclosed by the loss of alignment of the spinolaminar line at that level.

### Opacity:

- osteophyte
- opaque vertebral body from a sclerotic metastatic deposit (prostate and breast carcinoma) or from Paget's disease

### Radiolucency:

- fracture line
- spondylolysis
- gas in the disc

### Distortion or displacement:

- narrowed disc space
- compression fracture
- scoliosis
- spondylolisthesis
- retrolisthesis

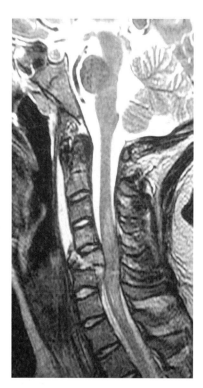

**Fig. 5.27** T2-weighted image. A fracture/dislocation at C5–6 in this 13-year-old girl who fell from a horse. Look carefully at the spinal cord to see the area of increased signal (whiter than normal) in the region of the fracture. This is a contusion of the cord. The disruption of the intervertebral disc is seen in a way that no other imaging can match. In the head identify the cerebellum, the fourth ventricle, the midbrain, pons and medulla, the basilar artery, the pituitary gland, and above it the optic chiasm.

### Frontal view

#### Where to look

Start in the middle

(1) spinous processes

(2) pedicles

(3) vertebral bodies

(4) intervertebral discs

(5) transverse processes

(6) paravertebral soft tissues

(7) sacroiliac (SI) joints

(8) check the arcuate lines of the sacrum

### Some diseases of the spine

Except for the prevertebral soft tissues and the disc spaces, all attention is directed to the bones.

Much of the information about disc disease comes from indirect information supplied by the bone changes and the relationships of the vertebrae to each other. Two disc diseases are important:

1. *Degenerative disc disease*, also called spondylosis, is a common cause of much suffering. The X-ray changes reflect the underlying pathogenesis. Defects develop in the annulus fibrosus and some of the nucleus pulposus prolapses in any radial direction, lifting the capsule and stimulating a periosteal reaction that causes an osteophyte. Larger prolapses if they occur posteriorly can compress a nerve in the spinal canal, this pathology requires a CT, MRI, or myelogram for imaging. Prolapse of nucleus material also occurs through the end plate and into the vertebral body, particularly when osteoporosis is present. More severe changes lead to a loss of fluid in the disc with consequent loss of disc height and later the formation of gas in the nucleus pulposus, visible in a plain film.

2. *Discitis*, is an uncommon infection caused by bacteria and recognized by erosion of the end plates above and below the disc.

Three joints, the disc and two apophyseal joints, connect the vertebrae to each other. In the apophyseal joints sclerosis of the subchondral bone and loss of articular cartilage with narrowing of the joint space are again the hallmarks of degenerative disease.

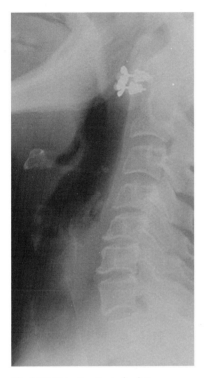

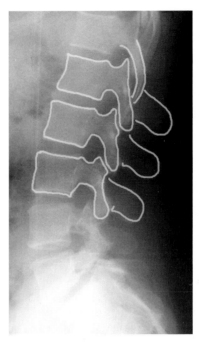

Fig. 5.29 Lateral view of the lumbar spine.

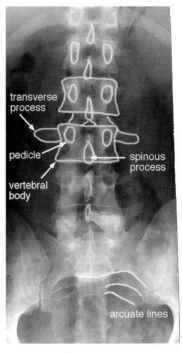

Fig. 5.30 Frontal view of the lumbar spine. The spinous process is the nose, the pedicles the eyes, the vertebral body the head, and the transverse processes the ears of a funny looking character.

Fig. 5.28 This place in the book is a reasonable opportunity to consider the soft tissues of the neck. An X-ray can be useful when a radio-opaque object such as a chicken or meat bone has been swallowed. In cases of fish bones it is of little use as they are often radiolucent. Sometimes an X-ray is ordered for acute epiglottitis. However this is a life-threatening disease and is best treated on clinical grounds even though an X-ray may confirm the diagnosis. The X-ray department is not the place to treat a respiratory arrest. To understand the anatomy look first for the hyoid bone. It bisects the epiglottis. Anterior to the epiglottis is the vallecula where foreign bodies often lodge. Usually in adults there is a variable degree of calcification of the thyroid and cricoid cartilages, which makes it difficult to distinguish foreign bodies. The arytenoids sit on the cricoid cartilage posteriorly, and from there the vocal cords pass forwards. Above the true cords is a dark area caused by air in the ventricle which separates the false cords above from the true cords below. Narrowing of the disc space and osteophyte formation indicates degenerative disease of the C4–5, C5–6, and C6–7 intervertebral discs. Studs mark the position of the ear lobes.

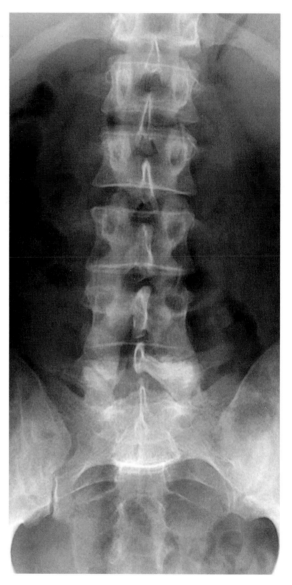

**Fig. 5.31** Five lumbar vertebrae. Mild scoliosis convex to the right. Scoliosis is a curvature of the spine in the coronal plane and may be accompanied by a rotational component. Idiopathic causes in which the bones are normal cause 70% of cases; 10% are due to congenital abnormalities of the vertebrae, and the remainder are a result of pain, trauma, neuromuscular, infectious, and neoplastic causes or simply having one leg longer than the other. The spinous processes are normal. Checking the pedicles reveals sclerosis on the left at L5, and on the right is an abnormal orientation of the apophyseal joint. The L5 lamina on the right side is not fused. This is one of the minor lumbosacral variants that are usually asymptomatic. In this case, the sclerosis on the left is probably a result of degenerative changes in the apophyseal joint. The vertebral bodies, disc spaces, sacroiliac joints, and the three arcuate lines of the sacrum are normal.

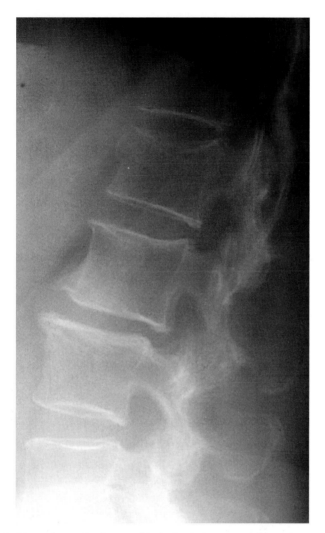

**Fig. 5.32** Looking at the *anterior alignment* of the bodies discloses several abnormalities:
- irregularity of the cortex of L1;
- osteophytes at L2–3;
- retrolisthesis of L2 on L3.

The *vertebral bodies* are abnormally radiolucent and the cortex is thinned, giving a 'picture frame' or 'empty box' appearance. T12 is recognized by the last rib. The bodies of T12 and L1 are distorted by wedge fractures. These are the appearances of osteoporosis and crush fractures from a flexion injury, deceleration in a motor vehicle accident. A third pathology is present, degenerative disease in the L2–3 disc. The signs which allow this diagnosis are: narrowing of the *disc space*, osteophyte formation, and retrolisthesis (posterior subluxation) of L2 on L3. Is the retrolisthesis caused by the trauma or by the spondylosis? In other words, was it present before the accident? More information would help. MRI or a CT myelogram can assess the degree of narrowing of the spinal canal.

### Hint

Have a look at an articulated skeleton occasionally to compare an X-ray to the 3D reality. It will be rewarding.

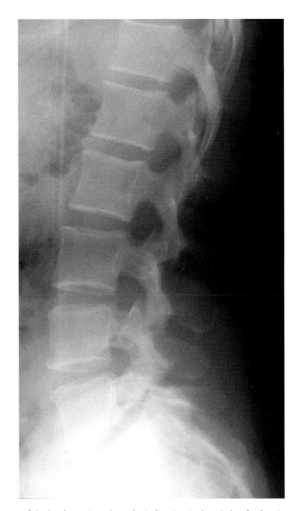

**Fig. 5.33** X-rays of the lumbar spine where the indication is chronic low back pain and no motor or sphincter disturbance should be performed sparingly, as degenerative disease is common and the X-ray changes may not correlate with the clinical picture. Imaging is needed if there are clinical indications of infection, tumour, spondylolisthesis, or ankylosing spondylitis. *Prevertebral tissues*: nothing significant *Anterior alignment*: Some small osteophytes distort the normal smooth, rounded corners of the *vertebral bodies* and signify early degenerative changes. *Disc spaces*: These appear unremarkable. *Posterior alignment* of the bodies: There is a forward slip of L5 on S1. The *pars interarticulares* of L5 show the defect of spondylolysis (footnote 16), a type of stress fracture of the bone between the superior and inferior articular facets. If the tips of the *spinous processes* are followed there is a step at the L4–L5 level, signifying forward slip of the body of L5, leaving its spinous process behind: spondylolisthesis.

16. spondylolysis from the Greek *spondylos* = vertebra and *lysis* = dissolution; spondylolisthesis = forward displacement of one vertebra on another, usually L5 on S1, sometimes L4 on L5; spondylosis = degenerative changes in the vertebral column due to osteoarthrosis.

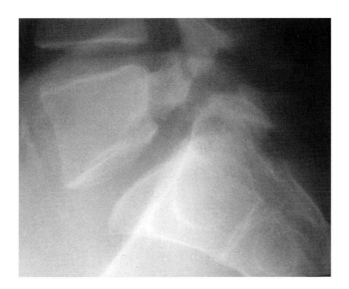

Fig. 5.34 A spot view showing spondylolysis of the pars interarticulares of L5 and the corresponding intact feature of the vertebra above. The lateral projection will usually show spondylolysis if it is present. The oblique view with the 'Scottie dog' appearance is no longer indicated as it adds considerably to the radiation dose and is unreliable in demonstrating a pars defect. If in doubt, ask for a CT.

*Hint*

Try not to miss any opportunity to show X-rays to a patient and explain the findings *slowly* and in simple terms. Ask if that makes it clearer, and you will be convinced that sometimes a picture is worth a thousand words.

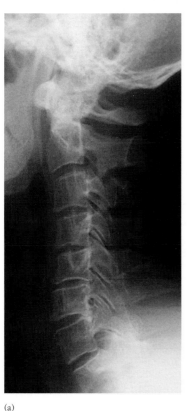

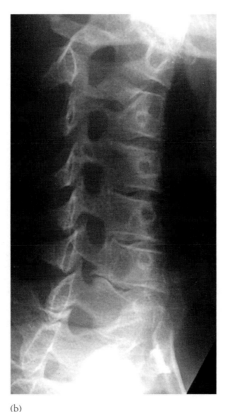

Figs 5.35 (a), (b) A 40-year-old man with neck pain and mild right hand paraesthesia. As there was no response to 6 weeks of conservative therapy, an X-ray was ordered. *Prevertebral soft tissues*: These are normal, as is the alignment of the *anterior surfaces* of the *vertebral bodies*. *Disc space*: The C5–6 intervertebral disc space is narrowed as is the C6–7 disc posteriorly. These are the changes of degenerative disease of the spine, cervical spondylosis, and could be secondary to previous trauma in someone of this age. *Posterior alignment*, *apophyseal joints*, and *spinous processes*: normal. The symptom was of paraesthesia in the right hand. The oblique view shows how osteophyte formation narrows the intervertebral foramen. Fibrous tissue of the intervertebral joint covers the osteophyte and makes the foramen even smaller than it appears here. The foramen on the other side had a similar appearance but there were no symptoms on that side. The radiological appearances must always be interpreted in the light of the clinical situation. MRI is probably a better investigation when brachalgia is present.

(a)                    (b)

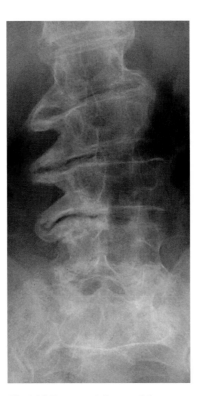

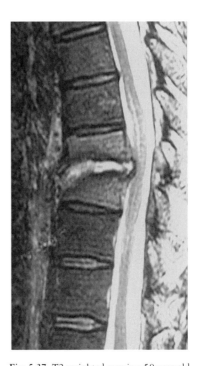

**Fig. 5.36** Pronounced changes of degenerative disc disease. Large osteophytes, narrowing of the disc spaces on the right side with consequent scoliosis. The radiolucency on the right side in the lower discs is gas formation. A space is formed in the degenerate disc because of shrinkage with desiccation. Normally the body would fill the space with granulation tissue and then scar tissue but as the nucleus pulposis has no blood supply this does not occur. Gas, mainly nitrogen, enters the space to equalize the pressure. Nature abhors a vacuum.

**Fig. 5.37** T2-weighted scan in a 50-year-old man. He had backache for 2 months and now was developing long tract signs. As you can imagine, the plain X-ray of the thoracic spine showed loss of the adjacent end plates (cortex) of the affected vertebral bodies. The MRI shows this destruction of the end plates, the inflammation and oedema in the disc space, the involvement of the vertebral bodies with osteomyelitis and partial collapse, and the extrusion of disc material into the spinal canal. All a result of discitis (infection of the disc). Beware of long tract signs. They slip past your guard because the patients may have little pain, just some weakness, and numbness of the legs and sphincter disturbances. They could be a result of disc prolapse, discitis, epidural abscess, or primary or secondary neoplasm.

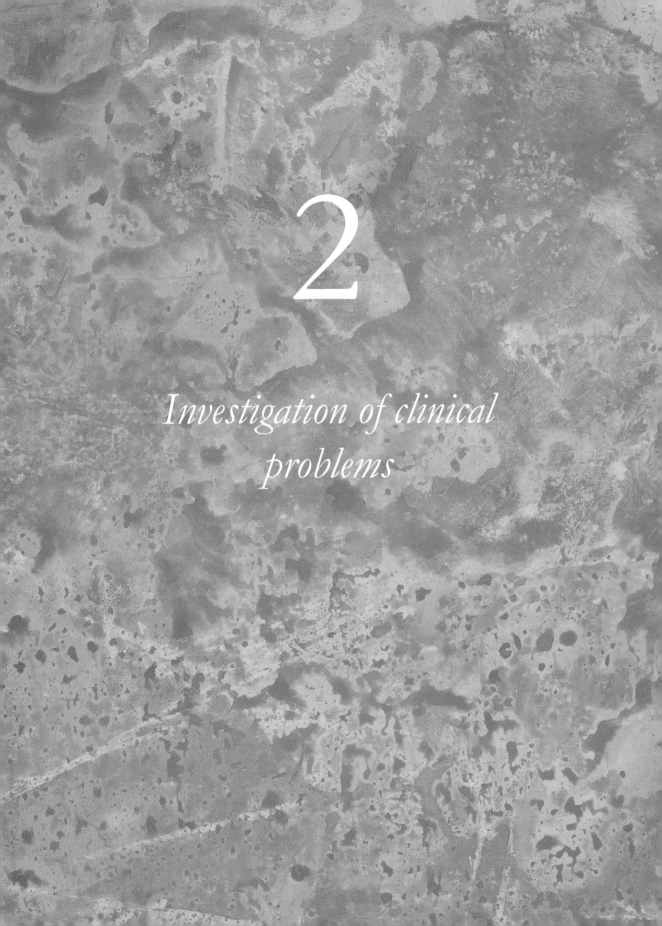

# 2

*Investigation of clinical problems*

It is not much use giving a first class interpretation of a chest or abdomen X-ray if the wrong investigation has been ordered.

This section looks at the investigation of a few specific problems in the body systems and indicates which imaging investigation is appropriate.

You may wonder why only 23 clinical situations are displayed when there must be more than a million ways that a patient may present.

They have been selected because they:

- are common or important conditions;

- demonstrate a particular imaging investigation;

- teach important thought processes, a logical thinking pattern.

Just as the first section of this book has a simple concept for where to look and what to look for, this section has an outline of *one* way that diagnostic thinking may best proceed.

When trying to work out the diagnosis and appropriate management the steps go something like this: Take the initial history and

1. Formulate a hypothesis of what is the problem, often a provisional diagnosis or differential diagnosis.

2. Perform the clinical examination. This is the first test. It is used to: *confirm* or *exclude* the diagnosis, *define* some feature or extent of pathology, or follow the *progress of* a known disease.

3. Act now if you have enough information.

4. If there is not enough information, you may order a pathology or imaging test to: confirm, exclude, define, or follow the progress of the suspected disease.

5. Act now if you have enough information.

6. If there is not enough information, consider ordering another pathology or imaging test to: confirm, exclude, define, or follow the progress of a disease.

7. Act now if you have enough information.

8. If there is still not enough information, before ordering another test consider rethinking the problem or organizing a second opinion.

The scenarios that follow use this approach.

Each case has a format of four questions that can be used in clinical situations:

1. What is the working diagnosis or differential diagnosis? 'Hypothesis' may be a better term as it is more general, encompassing conventional diagnoses as well as psychological and social issues and administrative demands.

2. What do I need to know?

3. Which imaging modality will confirm, exclude, define, or show the progress of this?

4. What may be shown and where do I go to from here? In particular, what will I do if the imaging appears normal?

Beginners find that thinking ahead to a variety of possible outcomes is a challenge. It is at first. The more astute the clinician, the better grasp she has of these concepts of likelihoods and outcomes.

The decision pathway is not presented as an algorithm since that format is probably not conducive to learning except for those who construct it. The selection of imaging tests is flexible. It will differ according to local custom and the availability of modalities.

One of the secrets of learning is to start with the core facts or principles and add other bits by association. The following outlines of investigation of problems is concise but hopefully provides a framework on which to add knowledge. Sometimes deciding which investigation to use is a complex decision. Full-time workers in the field (radiologists) have more experience and know more of the minutiae. Consult them as needed.

What you can learn from this section:

- pathways of thoughtful, logical, and cost-effective investigation of clinical problems;

- information about different imaging modalities: uses, preparation, advantages, disadvantages, and contraindications;

- appearances of important disorders;

- better understanding of the radiology reports of complex imaging.

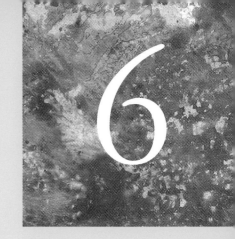

# 6

# *Investigation of the respiratory system*

- Cases 1, 2, and 3:

  What is the working diagnosis or differential diagnosis?

  What do I need to know?

  Which imaging modality will confirm, exclude, define, or show the progress of this?

  What may be shown, and where do I go from here?

## Case 1

A 30-year-old male has been brought to the emergency department following a high-speed motor vehicle accident. He is unconscious and has multiple abrasions, several on the chest wall. The abdomen is soft. BP is 90/50. Pulse is 120, same as yours. He has been intubated and two IV lines are in. You remember that the three most important X-rays are the lateral cervical spine, chest, and pelvis and order all three. Now is the time to put into practice your radiological skills. All the routine films you have seen have been practice for this occasion of life-and-death decisions under the pressure of time and accuracy. The C-spine and pelvis films are normal.

## What is the working diagnosis or differential diagnosis?

Chest trauma

## What do I need to know?

- Is there any blood or gas where they should not be?
- Is the cardiac silhouette enlarged?
- Is the diaphragm intact?
- Any fractures?

## Which imaging modality will confirm, exclude, define, or show the progress of this?

Chest X-ray

## CXR

*Description:*
- A CXR demonstrates the morphology of the chest reasonably well. It projects the three-dimensional chest onto a two-dimensional film or monitor screen. Technical steps are taken to show the lungs and diminish the prominence of the ribs. It does not of course show function, but some changes can indicate a restrictive lung disease (small lung volumes) or an obstructive one (bullae and hyperexpansion of emphysema).

## CXR (continued)

- The CXR is usually a *supine* film in seriously ill people, which means that fluid will layer posteriorly, a pneumothorax will lie anteriorly, lung volumes will appear decreased except if ventilated, and the mediastinal structures will be wider than in a PA film.

### Patient preparation:

- nil

### Advantages:

- It is cheap and quick, good for imaging the lungs, pleural spaces, and diaphragm.

### Disadvantages:

- CXR is a coarse indicator of mediastinal disease, a place where CT is much better at demonstrating the anatomy and pathology.

### Contraindications:

- Take care with females who may be pregnant; nil for others. The sicker someone is, the more they need a CXR.

## What may be shown, and where do I go from here?

### What if it is normal?

Think of other explanations for hypotension and tachycardia. A normal chest X-ray does not exclude every type of aortic injury.

### What if it is abnormal?

This is a great example of the use of a systematic review of a radiograph because almost any change can occur and must be sought.

- A pneumothorax will need an intercostal catheter.

- A widened mediastinum in a stable patient requires a CT and/or an aortogram to confirm or exclude the presence of blood, aortic rupture, pericardial blood. There is no simple measurement to say what is a widened mediastinum. If you are *not sure*, please do not say to a colleague, 'I think the mediastinum is widened. What do you think?' Say, 'Is the mediastinum widened?' The first statement has the effect of placing undue pressure on the clinician to run an extensive battery of tests to exclude serious illness.

- An elevated hemidiaphragm, particularly on the left, may indicate rupture, the right side being protected by the liver. Raise the possibility with a senior colleague. It is a difficult diagnosis to confirm or exclude.

- Fractures of the ribs, sternum, shoulder girdle, and spine may need other views or imaging modalities.

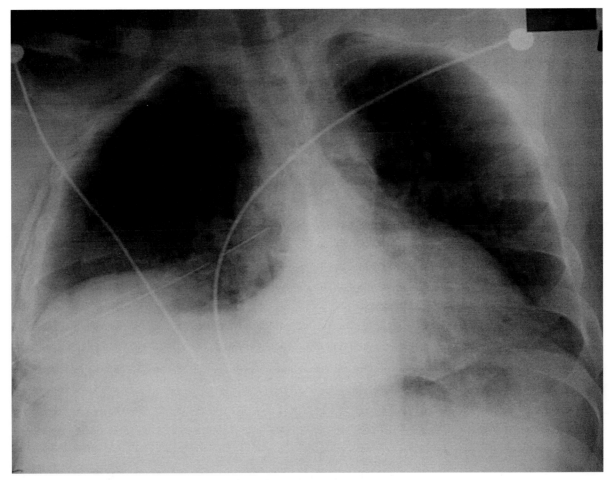

**Fig. 6.1** The radiographs of people who are sick, particularly *really* sick, are often not perfect but may be the best obtainable at the time. Instead of criticizing the film, get what you can from it. Check the position of the tubes and lines first. An intercostal catheter has already been inserted. It looks well positioned but could lie in the oblique fissure, the subcutaneous tissues, or in the bed, limiting its effectiveness. If it is not working put in a new one or organize a CT to see where it is. The ECG monitoring leads are seen. *Lungs*: the upper zone of the right hemithorax is radiolucent. *Pleura*: The pleural edge of the collapsed right lung is seen. That means that the lung has not had enough time to re-expand or that the tube is blocked. *Mediastinum*: This is shifted a little to the left. *Hila*: difficult to see. *Bones*: When looking at the bones do not miss the fractured clavicle. *Soft tissues*: Subcutaneous gas is present in the soft tissues because of the rib fractures and insertion of the tube. The right hemidiaphragm is elevated. This could be from the pain of a rib fracture or some pathology in the abdomen.

## Case 2

A 42-year-old woman has noticed right-sided chest pain for the last 12 hours. The pain is worse on inspiration, giving a sensation of not allowing a full inspiration, but is not associated with a cough or fever. She had surgery for carcinoma of the cervix 9 days previously, is overweight, has mild cardiac failure from chemotherapy, and has a history of a pulmonary embolus. At the moment, she is neither pregnant nor taking oral contraceptives.

### What is the working diagnosis or differential diagnosis?

Pulmonary embolism with lung infarction (pleuritic pain) rather than haemorrhage (haemoptysis)

### What do I need to know?

This is a pleuritic pain. One needs to know if it is caused by primary pleurisy or irritation of the pleura by pneumonia, lung infarction, or a pneumothorax.

### Which imaging modality will *confirm*, exclude, define, or show the progress of this?

CXR

### What may be shown, and where do I go from here?

*What if it is normal?*

A normal CXR does not exclude pulmonary embolism. Whether the probability is low, medium, or high a further test is needed to confirm or exclude the disease.

*What if it is abnormal?*

The usefulness of the CXR is in showing:
- pleural fluid secondary to pleuritis;
- consolidation in the lung, caused by infection or haemorrhage;
- a pneumothorax;
- a wedge-shaped peripheral opacity of pulmonary infarction.

The CXR turns out to be almost normal. It does not explain the symptoms and cannot exclude a pulmonary embolus. Move to Phase 2.

### What do I need to know?

Is there a pulmonary embolus or another cause of pleuritic pain?

### Which imaging modality will *confirm*, exclude, define, or show the progress of this?

A CT pulmonary angiogram
A radionuclear ventilation/perfusion (V/Q) lung scan

# CT pulmonary angiogram

## Description and uses:

- This study replaces the radionuclear V/Q scan in many centres. It is made possible by helical scanners that have formidable X-ray tubes capable of high heat capacity. 100 slices are taken in one breath-hold (30 s) while injecting contrast rapidly (100 ml at 4 ml/s). The lumen of the pulmonary arteries is seen down to the fifth order (fourth bifurcation) or more.

## Patient preparation:

- Be kind to a radiologist. Insert a large bore, 18- or 20-gauge IV cannula for administering the contrast.

## Advantages:

- It is fast, can be completed in 20 minutes; has high sensitivity and specificity; and detects other pathologies.

## Disadvantages:

- Contrast reactions.

## Contraindications:

- Allergy to contrast media.
- Most other relative contraindications are outweighed by the importance of the information sought, is there a clot or not?

# What may be shown, and where do I go from here?

## What if it is normal?

A pulmonary embolus is effectively excluded, although some centres may wish to perform a pulmonary angiogram.

## What if it is abnormal?

- filling defect in the pulmonary artery indicating an embolus;
- collapse or consolidation;
- pleural effusion;
- pneumothorax;
- aortic dissection.

Treatment can usually be commenced with these results.

**Fig. 6.2** The main pulmonary artery travels posteriorly and divides into the right and left arteries. Large clots are seen in these two branches. The IV contrast shows as white. This CT slice is at the level of the hila. Anterior to the clot in the right pulmonary artery are three vessels: the smallest is the superior pulmonary vein coming down to join the left atrium a little more inferiorly; next is the oval shape of the superior vena cava; and the largest is the ascending aorta. The density of the hilum on a chest X-ray is formed by the pulmonary artery and superior pulmonary vein. On the left side, anterior to the left main bronchus is the superior pulmonary vein. The left pulmonary artery has arched over the bronchus and that is why the left hilum is a centimetre higher than that on the right. The descending pulmonary artery is filled with clot. The oesophagus contains some gas and lies anterior to the descending aorta.

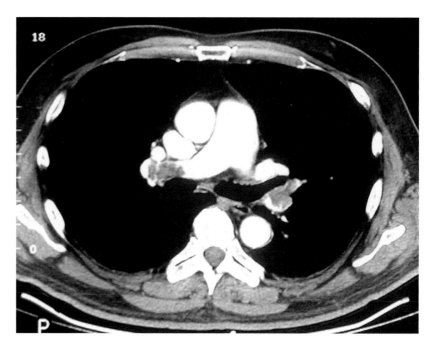

# Case 3

> A 42-year-old woman has been in intensive care, on a respirator for 5 days follow-
> ing abdominal sepsis and a laparotomy. You, as the resident on duty, notice that her
> pulse rate has increased, the ventilation pressures are rising, and her blood pressure
> is falling.

## What is the working diagnosis or differential diagnosis?

A problem with lung compliance

## What do I need to know?

Is this a problem of the tubes, airway, lung, or pleural space?

## Which imaging modality will confirm, exclude, define, or show the progress of this?

CXR

## What may be shown, and where do I go from here?

### What if it is normal or at least not changed?

Look for some problem outside the lungs, causing elevated pressures. Is the
endotracheal tube kinked? Is there increased intra-abdominal pressure? Is the
patient undersedated and breathing asynchronously with the respirator?

### What if it is abnormal?

- lung collapse from mucous plugging;
- acute respiratory distress syndrome (ARDS)—formerly known as the adult
  respiratory distress syndrome, a disorder of capillary damage in the lungs;
- pneumothorax;
- large pleural effusion.

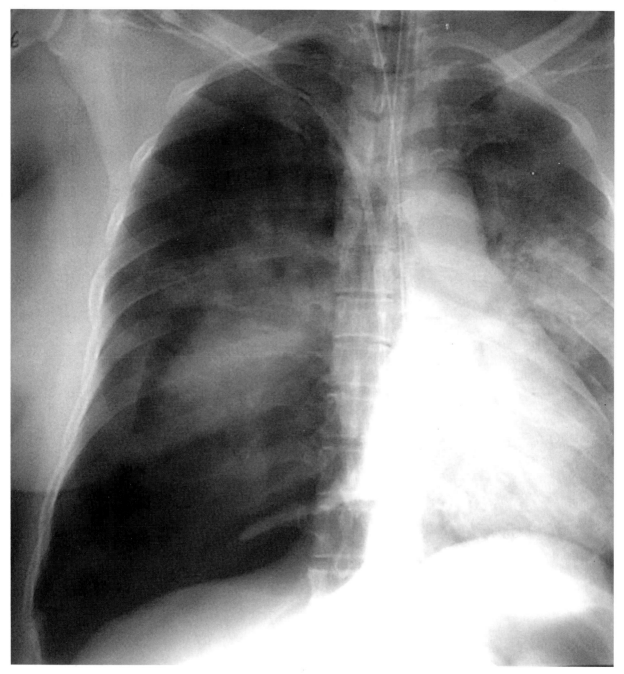

**Fig. 6.3** This is a great educational film from the intensive care unit. The inexperienced doctor could be distracted by the poor quality, badly centred film. The technicians do the best they can under difficult conditions. To ask for another film in this instance would be a mistake. There is adequate information to make a life-saving decision. After checking the name of the patient, see that the tubes and lines are well positioned: the endotracheal and nasogastric tubes and the right subclavian central venous line. *Lungs*: The left lung shows consolidation. The right hemithorax is too black and hyperexpanded. Right hemidiaphragm is depressed. *Pleura*: The pleural recess is seen at the right base. *Mediastinum*: This is shifted to the left, obstructing venous return and decreasing cardiac output, a threat to life. Is it being pushed or pulled? *Hila, bones,* and *soft tissues*: Check these structures. Is the endotracheal tube down the right main bronchus, inflating the right lung and collapsing the left? No. Is the right lung collapsed? Yes. Right tension pneumothorax. Beware of the half-toning of the hemidiaphragm in a supine film. In the supine position, a pneumothorax will be anterior and the lung will fall posteriorly. A chest tube is needed immediately. The consolidation in the left lung could be a result of any of the causes of the acute respiratory distress syndrome (ARDS). Consolidation/collapse often occurs in intubated patients at the left base. Suction catheters to clear the lungs pass down the ETT and preferentially into the right main bronchus.

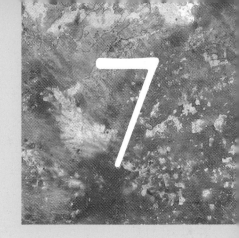

7

# Investigation of the cardiovascular system

- Cases 1 and 2:

  *What is the working diagnosis or differential diagnosis?*

  *What do I need to know?*

  *Which imaging modality will confirm, exclude, define, or show the progress of this?*

  *What may be shown, and where do I go from here?*

## Case 1

A 75-year-old male patient has a history of increasing claudication in the left leg. He has been smoking since the war. Who could blame him, long periods of boredom and exercises sprinkled with episodes of terror. Interestingly, he had stopped smoking 2 years ago when you had advised him to do it. It had given you hope at the time—someone actually is listening to your advice.

Over the last 10 months, the pain in the calf has worsened and now he can only walk 75 metres on level ground before having to stop for a rest.

Examination reveals moderate pulses in the right leg and a moderate femoral pulse on the left. The distal pulses in the left leg are absent.

## What is the working diagnosis or differential diagnosis?

Severe stenosis or occlusion of the left superficial femoral artery

## What do I need to know?

- Where is the stenosis?
- What is the state of the distal run-off?
- Is there a significant vessel that a graft can be attached to?
- Is there a localized stenosis suitable for treatment with angioplasty, (footnote 17) expansion of a balloon in the lumen?

## Which imaging modality will confirm, exclude, *define*, or show the progress of this?

An aortobifemoral angiogram

## What may be shown, and where do I go from here?
### *What if it is normal?*

Highly unlikely, but stranger things have happened! If the patient was obese and had previous surgery to the popliteal fossa, the pulse may have been difficult to appreciate. Once the popliteal pulse was not felt perhaps the others were

---

17.    plasty = a suffix indicating plastic surgery, repair, remodelling, moulding.

## Aortobifemoral angiogram

### Description and uses:

- A catheter is inserted usually into the right common femoral artery and advanced to the distal aorta. Contrast is injected and AP and oblique views are taken. It shows the diameter of the lumen, stenoses, obstruction, collateral flow, vessel re-formation, and gives an estimate of the flow rate.

### Patient preparation:

- 'Fluids only' for 4 hours prior to the procedure.
- Premedication is not essential but some patients may prefer it.
- Obtain informed consent.

### Advantages:

- It gives a clear 2D image of the 3D arterial tree.

### Disadvantages:

- As with all angiograms, the contrast shows only the lumen.
- Aneurysms with clot may be underestimated.
- Contrast reactions
- Damage to the arteries
- Large doses of contrast may impair the kidneys.
- Bleeding from the puncture site.

### Contraindications:

- Allergy to contrast.
- Pregnancy, usually only applicable with trauma victims, and even then one may have to proceed but with a modified technique.

missed, because one expected that they would not be there. Think of other possible diagnoses such as spinal stenosis.

### What if it is abnormal?

- Stenosis or obstruction of the superficial femoral artery.

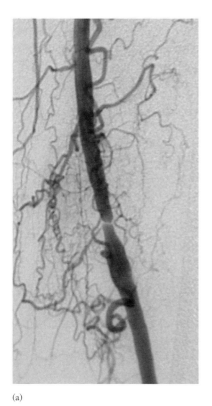

(a)

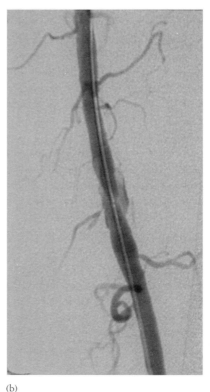

(b)

**Figs** 7.1 (a), (b) The pre-angioplasty film shows a 90% stenosis of the superficial femoral artery. The collateral flow indicates it is a significant stenosis and has been present for some time. Clinically there was a significant obstruction. Often the disease is not localized like this and a femoropopliteal graft would be needed. In this case, an angioplasty was performed to dilate the short stenosis. The expansion of the balloon has caused disruption of the plaque.

## Case 2

A 60-year-old man had a right total hip replacement 10 days before he came to see you with a history of swelling of the right leg over the previous 2 days. He is on treatment for cardiac failure and 3 years ago had a carcinoma of the colon removed. The two other aspects of history taking have not been neglected: placing the disease in the context of his lifestyle; and establishing a rapport that ensures mutual understanding and patient cooperation with the agreed plan of management. Examination reveals a swollen thigh and calf. You are mindful of the difficulty of diagnosing a deep vein thrombosis (DVT), 50% of them showing no clinical signs and only 30% of those who have clinical signs having a proven DVT.

## What is the working diagnosis or differential diagnosis?

DVT

## What do I need to know?

The presence and extent of the clot. Thrombi in the calf have much less chance of producing an embolus than those in the thigh and pelvis.

Which imaging modality will *confirm*, exclude, define, or show the progress of this?

A duplex (meaning double, images and flow) ultrasound examination is cheaper and safer than a venogram and is the investigation of choice.

## Ultrasound scan

*Description and uses:*

- The clot discloses its presence by obstructing flow, shown by colour Doppler, and by its incompressibility.
- Normal vein walls can be apposed by pressure from the ultrasound probe, best seen in the transverse view.

*Disadvantages:*

- Some parts of the deep venous system may be difficult to visualize if the leg is swollen.

## Venogram

*Description and uses:*

- 50 ml of contrast is injected into a vein on the dorsum of the foot. Radiographs will demonstrate if there is a filling defect or occlusion of a vein caused by a thrombus.

*Patient preparation:*

- Obtain informed consent.

*Advantages:*

- This is useful when the ultrasound is technically difficult or indeterminate. It will show the external and common iliac veins in the pelvis and also the calf veins, areas where ultrasound has difficulty.

*Disadvantages:*

- There is a 1 in 100 000 risk of death with a contrast injection.

*Contraindications:*

- Allergy to contrast
- Pregnancy

What may be shown, and where do I go from here?

*What if it is normal?*

Have the veins of the pelvis been seen satisfactorily? Is it cellulitis/infection, injury, superficial phlebitis?

## *What if it is abnormal?*

- A thrombus requires treatment.

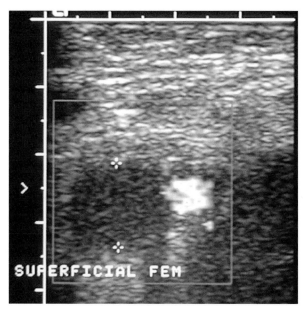

**Fig. 7.2** This is an ultrasound study with engagement of the Doppler mode. It shows the bright area which indicates flow in the superficial femoral artery. It would be red or blue on the screen or in a colour photograph. Red, by convention, indicates flow towards the transducer and blue signifies flow going away. The vein has a much larger diameter than the artery. This occurs with thrombosis because the blood flows around between the clot and the wall, gradually increasing the size of the clot. The chief indicator of a deep vein thrombus is incompressibility of the vessel. The vessel walls were not able to be approximated with pressure from the transducer at the time of the examination.

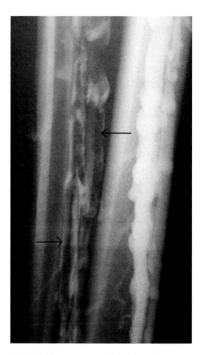

**Fig. 7.3** A venogram of the right calf. Thrombus almost fills the two peroneal veins that accompany the artery. The contrast flows around the clot which is classed as a 'filling defect'.

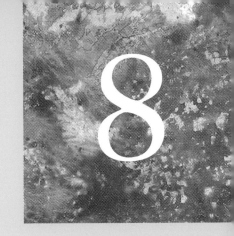

# 8

# Investigation of the gastrointestinal tract

- Cases 1–6:

  What is the working diagnosis or differential diagnosis?

  What do I need to know?

  Which imaging modality will confirm, exclude, define, or show the progress of this?

  What may be shown, and where do I go from here?

# Investigation of the gastrointestinal tract

## Case 1

> A 45-year-old woman comes to see you. As she walks through the door, the generic diagnosis is apparent. Her sclerae are yellow.
> Examination is otherwise unremarkable.
> Hepatitis serology is negative.

### What is the working diagnosis or differential diagnosis?

Obstructive or non-obstructive jaundice

### What do I need to know?

- Is there an obstruction and if so where is the site?
- Does the liver look normal?

### Which imaging modality will confirm, exclude, *define*, or show the progress of this?

Ultrasound

## Ultrasound

*Patient preparation:*
- fasting for 8 hours to fill the gall-bladder

*Contraindications:*
- nil

### What may be shown, and where do I go from here?

*What if it is normal?*

The common duct can be of normal calibre (<6 mm diameter), suggesting a pre-hepatic or hepatic cause of jaundice. Perhaps it is obstructed and has not had time to dilate. A liver biopsy may be required.

*What if it is abnormal?*

- Dilated ducts—the obstruction can be:
  - *luminal*: choledocholithiasis—ultrasound will detect 40% of common duct stones (Abboud *et al*. 1996);
  - *mural*: stricture following cholecystectomy;
  - *extramural*: acute or chronic pancreatitis, carcinoma of the head of the pancreas.

  **Note**: Dilated ducts can occur without obstruction in the elderly and in people who previously had common duct stones.

- Liver diseases that cause jaundice can sometimes be demonstrated.
- Ultrasound can show related pathology such as stones in the gall-bladder, acute or chronic cholecystitis, and primary tumour of the gall-bladder.

May need to proceed to:

- CT: demonstrates extramural masses and distant spread of carcinoma;
- ERCP (endoscopic retrograde cholangiopancreatography) and MRI cholangiography: will show stones, strictures, inflammation, and tumours of the biliary tree.

**Fig. 8.1** The three vessels in the porta hepatis are shown here. The sonographer will label the structures to allow recognition on the hard or soft copy because it is not easy to interpret ultrasound images without guidance. The label here is bile duct, long (itudinal scan). It cannot be called the common hepatic duct or the common bile duct because one cannot usually see where the cystic duct joins and defines this name change. Deep to the bile duct and running parallel is the portal vein. The right hepatic artery curves between the two and is seen in cross-section as a black circle. The cursors measure the duct diameter as 8 mm, too big. A cause should be found. Is there an obstruction at present: intraluminal, mural, or extramural? Was there an obstruction in the past, leaving the duct dilated?

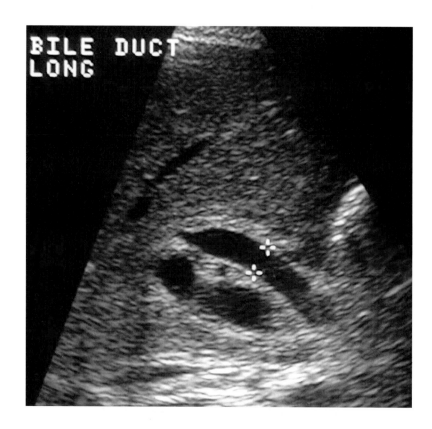

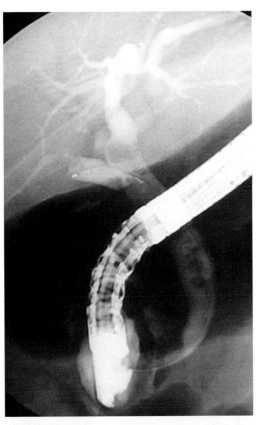

**Fig. 8.2** ERCP is a useful investigation. It allows both diagnosis of a calculus or other obstruction as well as some treatment options: the removal of a calculus, sphincterotomy (of the sphincter of Oddi) to drain the system or allow passage of a calculus, and stenting (passing a tube to keep the lumen open). The filling defects are stones in the common duct. Over 80% of biliary tree calculi are radiolucent.

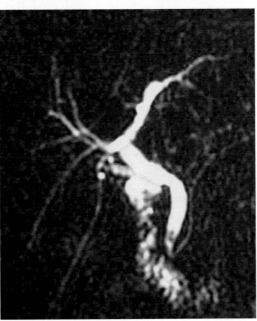

**Fig. 8.3** MR cholangiography is safer than an ERCP for imaging the biliary tree. Here it demonstrates a calculus in the distal common bile duct, just above the sphincter of Oddi.

## Case 2

A 60-year-old man comes to see you. His problem is one of difficulty with swallowing. Over the last month, food has been difficult to swallow but fluids are not such a problem.

## What is the working diagnosis or differential diagnosis?

Mechanical or functional (dysmotility) obstruction of the oesophagus

## What do I need to know?

The site and nature of the obstruction

## Which imaging modality will confirm, exclude, define, or show the progress of this?

A barium swallow or endoscopy

## Barium swallow

### Description and uses:

- Barium is usually the medium preferred because it is cheap and effective. A non-ionic contrast is used initially in cases where leakage, a fistula, or aspiration is suspected. The study reveals the anatomy of the upper digestive tract and also provides functional information, particularly when a video recording is made. Swallowing, peristalsis effectiveness, and gastro-oesophageal reflux can be shown.

### Patient preparation:

- Nothing to eat, drink, or smoke for 8 hours before the procedure.

### Advantages:

- Provides anatomical detail and some functional information.

### Disadvantages:

- It needs an endoscopy to follow when a biopsy is required.

### Contraindications:

- nil
- Take precautions with aspiration and pregnancy.

# What may be shown, and where do I go from here?

## What if it is normal?

Could it be an intermittent functional obstruction? Do you accept the negative test or proceed to an endoscopy? It depends on the pretest probability.

## What if it is abnormal

- Mechanical obstruction:
  - *luminal*: tumour, foreign body;
  - *mural*: stricture, tumour, oesophageal web, diverticulum;
  - *extramural*: compression by a neoplasm, nodes, goitre.
- Functional obstruction:
  - *presbyoesophagus*: degenerative changes occurring with ageing and causing uncoordinated peristalsis;
  - *achalasia*: a failure of the lower oesophageal sphincter to relax—it is accompanied by proximal dilatation;
  - *cerebrovascular accident*.

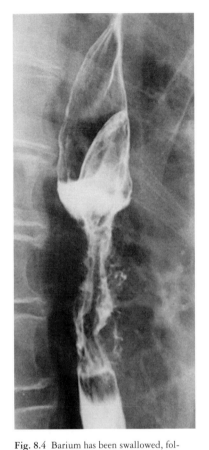

**Fig. 8.4** Barium has been swallowed, followed by some air. Over a length of a few centimetres the lumen is narrowed and the mucosa of the wall is quite irregular. This is an obstruction by an intramural lesion. It started as a single focus, spread by infiltrating the wall, encircling the lumen, and then extended cephalad and caudad. It probably extends into the mediastinal fat tissues because the serosa of the thoracic oesophagus is absent. It has caused ulceration of the mucosa and is almost certainly a carcinoma. A piece of food has been swallowed and was not able to pass. CT and transoesophageal ultrasound will allow the staging of a tumour. Seek any evidence of local spread or metastases to the nodes of the mediastinum and abdomen, or to the lung and liver

## Case 3

A 50-year-old man was painting his house when he fell from a ladder and landed across a tree stump. The paramedics who brought him by ambulance reported his BP as 120/80, PR 108. Abrasions are visible across the abdomen. He apparently has no other injuries.

The examination reveals a tender abdomen with guarding but no rigidity. Urine testing shows a trace of blood.

While in the emergency department a chest, lumbar spine, and pelvis X-rays were performed and were normal.

## What is the working diagnosis or differential diagnosis?

Trauma to the solid or hollow organs of the abdomen and pelvis

## What do I need to know?

Which organs are involved and to what extent?

## Spiral CT

### Description and uses:

- Spiral CT has added speed to an examination that clearly demonstrates the contents of the abdomen and pelvis as well as the abdominal wall.
- Oral contrast is usually given; IV contrast will be used to demonstrate the integrity of the liver, spleen, kidneys, and pancreas.

### Patient preparation:

- Oral contrast is given, if time is available for it to reach the colon or at least the small intestine.

### Advantages:

- High-resolution images are available in less than 30 minutes. With sick people who are moving and not breath-holding, unless anaesthetized, the images need considerable experience for appropriate interpretation.

### Disadvantages:

- It cannot be performed at the bedside like ultrasound.
- A substantial radiation dose is delivered.
- It needs contrast.

### Contraindications:

- Allergy to contrast.
- Care needed with pregnancy.

### Which imaging modality will confirm, exclude, *define*, or show the progress of this?

CT abdomen and pelvis in the stable patient. Unstable patients go directly to the operating theatre.

### What may be shown, and where do I go from here?

#### *What if it is normal?*

One would have to explain the tachycardia and haematuria. Perhaps they arise from pain and a kidney contusion. Contrast enhancement on CT should exclude avulsion of a kidney. Observation may be appropriate.

#### *What if it is abnormal?*

- blood in the peritoneal cavity, retroperitoneum, pleural spaces;
- laceration of the liver, spleen, kidney;
- gas in the retroperitoneum or peritoneal cavity.

With this information, a decision can be made as to operative intervention or conservative management.

A cystogram may need to be performed to confirm or exclude a bladder rupture.

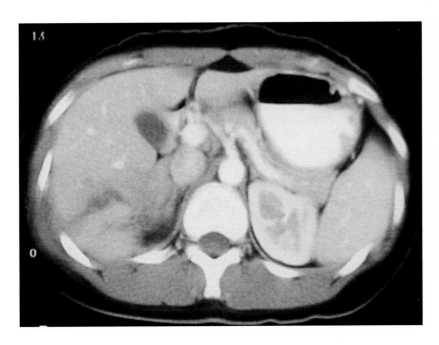

**Fig. 8.5** Intravenous contrast was injected. The contrast taken orally fills the stomach. The aorta is well opacified and the splenic artery can be seen behind the pancreas and heading towards the spleen. The hepatic artery curves to the right (of the patient) and passes anterior to the well-opacified portal vein seen in cross-section. To the right of this vein is the first part of the duodenum with contrast in the lumen. Between the duodenum and the liver is the low attenuation (black) of fluid in the gall-bladder. Posterior to the portal vein is the IVC. Perfusion of the left kidney seems adequate. The right kidney would be on a lower slice. The abnormality is in the right lobe of the liver, a linear area of low attenuation meaning no perfusion. This is a liver laceration with a haematoma. No free fluid is seen in the abdominal cavity so the liver capsule may be intact.

## Case 4

A 50-year-old woman has come to see you because of right upper quadrant discomfort, present for a week. You examine her abdomen and find that the liver edge is 6 cm below the costal margin. There is no evidence of jaundice.

## What is the working diagnosis or differential diagnosis?

Hepatomegaly

## Causes of hepatomegaly

- Rule out the common, diffuse conditions of hepatitis, infectious mononucleosis, right heart failure, fatty infiltration, and cirrhosis.
- Use ultrasound to confirm or exclude a mass, abscess, or cyst and look at the arterial and venous inflow and outflow.
- If no answer, check your favourite list of the 20+ causes.

## What do I need to know?

Is the liver diffusely enlarged, or is there a mass in or near the liver causing the findings on palpation?

## Which imaging modality will confirm, exclude, define, or show the progress of this?

Ultrasound or CT

## What may be shown, and where do I go from here?

### What if it is normal?

The liver shape varies considerably. Some people have a large right lobe of the liver and a small left lobe. This right lobe can extend to the iliac crest, simulating hepatomegaly, and is called a Riedel's lobe.

People with chronic obstructive airways disease have a low diaphragm. This will cause the edge of the liver to be palpable.

### What if it is abnormal?

The clinical assessment of hepatomegaly and splenomegaly is tricky. If it is an important clinical finding it may be best to confirm it with an ultrasound investigation.

- Diffuse enlargement of the liver
- A liver mass or masses:

  non-neoplastic such as:

  – *a cyst*: a simple cyst is usually best left alone—a hydatid cyst should go;

— *an abscess*: many organisms can cause hepatic abscesses—best known is the amoebic abscess produced by the protozoa *Entamoeba histolytica*;

neoplastic such as:

— *benign*: such as an haemangioma or focal nodular hyperplasia—MRI will help confirm the nature of these lesions;

— *malignant*, primary tumour: hepatocellular carcinoma;

— secondary: from many sources but particularly the colon.

- Extrahepatic mass.
- Associated pathology

ascites

splenomegaly

varices

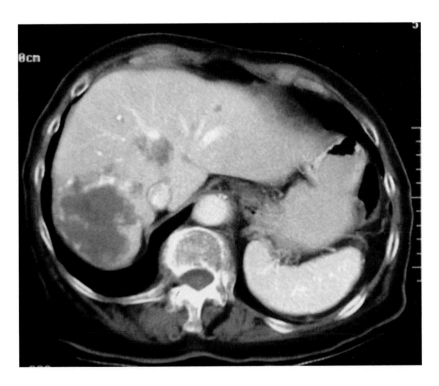

**Fig. 8.6** A CT examination after an injection of intravenous contrast. The poorly defined mass with irregular margins and satellite nodules is a fast-growing metastatic deposit probably with a necrotic centre. A fine-needle aspiration biopsy (FNAB) or excision biopsy can be performed to determine its nature, and perhaps the site of the primary tumour if that will affect the management.

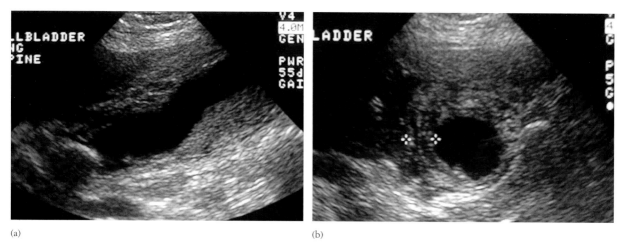

(a)　　　　　　　　　　　　　　　　　　　　　　　　　　(b)

**Figs 8.7** (a), (b)  Right upper quadrant pain in another person, someone quite ill. In the longitudinal view of the gall-bladder, the wall is not clearly demonstrated because of oedema and inflammation. The hypoechoic (black) area is bile in the gall-bladder. In the neck is the cresenteric, white reflection of the outline of the leading edge of a calculus. Sludge is present in the lumen, secondary to obstruction. Accompanying acute cholecystitis was indicated by three findings: thickening of the gall-bladder wall which measures 11 mm (normally <4 mm); pericholecystic fluid shown by the curvilinear, black stripes in and around the wall; and local tenderness of the gall-bladder at the time of the examination.

# Case 5

> The ambulance brings to the emergency department a 50-year-old man who has severe upper abdominal pain. Alcohol abuse has been a problem in the past. Examination reveals a tender epigastrium with guarding. A serum amylase reading is already back from the pathology department and is high.

## What is the working diagnosis or differential diagnosis?

Acute pancreatitis

## What do I need to know?

- What is the extent of the disease?
- Are there complications present: fluid collections (pseudocysts), ascites?

## Which imaging modality will *confirm*, exclude, define, or show the progress of this?

CT. MRI will give similar information to CT, but without the radiation.

## What may be shown, and where do I go from here?

### What if it is normal?

Perhaps the macroscopic changes of pancreatitis have not yet developed. Think of another pathology such as a penetrating peptic ulcer.

### What if it is abnormal?

- Signs of pancreatitis. The enzymes escape into the parenchyma and surrounding tissues, exactly why is unclear, but it probably has something to do with obstruction of the ducts. The CT appearances reflect the pathology: a swollen, oedematous pancreas with areas of haemorrhage and necrosis; peripancreatic fluid in the retroperitoneum and spreading into the mesentery; ascites; localized inflammatory fluid and tissue that may develop into a pseudocyst (footnote 18).
- The degree of pancreatic necrosis. Surgery may be indicated to debride the tissue. Follow up the development with CT scans.
- Causes such as gallstones, stones in the common bile duct (CBD) or calcification in the gland which would indicate chronic pancreatitis. Ultrasound is the best method of detecting gallstones in the gall-bladder. It will also show 40% of stones in the common bile duct or common hepatic duct.

---

18. Pancreatitis is a chemical burn to the abdomen and must be treated with respect. Sometimes some of this inflammatory fluid is walled off by the body's defences. The wall has no epithelial lining like true cysts, and therefore the collection is called a pseudocyst. It may need open or percutaneous drainage.

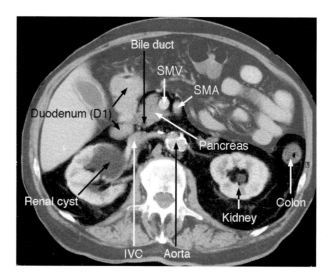

**Fig. 8.8** The retroperitoneum is quite extensive. It contains the kidneys, duodenum, pancreas, aorta, IVC, and ascending and descending colon.

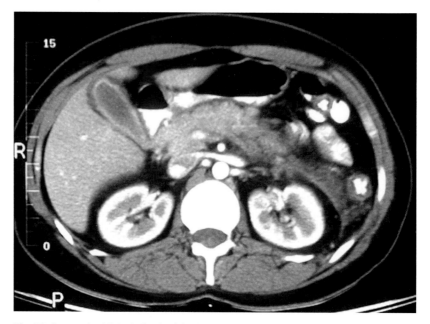

**Fig. 8.9** Once again, this is the key level for CT anatomy in the abdomen. Identify the liver, gall-bladder, first part of the duodenum, pancreas, SMV, and SMA. Behind the SMA is the left renal vein entering the IVC. Posterior to the left renal vein is the white, contrast-filled aorta and two renal arteries. There is oedema fluid around the pancreas and extending along the left anterior pararenal space to the descending colon (also a retroperitoneal structure). The inflammatory fluid also tracks up to the right, around the gall-bladder. The pancreas appears to be adequately perfused. This is a moderate degree of pancreatitis. Something has triggered a release of pancreatic enzymes into the parenchyma leaving this trail of tissue damage. Next step is to find the cause.

# Case 6

A young mother has brought in her 8-month-old child. The child looks unhappy but the mother... the mother has fear in her voice and guilt on her face as she tells you her story. It is half history, half apology. The child was sitting on the floor while the mother was sewing and was seen to put something in his mouth. His mother called to him and just at that moment he swallowed and started coughing. Had there been a pin on the floor?

A wise old doctor had told you about accidents in the home. How if children grow up without having a serious accident it is due to good management but with a generous serving of good luck. How the parents will feel intense guilt until recovery is complete.

At previous consultations you had formed the opinion that of all parents this woman was one who thought that children needed to be heard, hugged, protected, valued, nurtured, supported, complimented, encouraged, praised, admired, respected, cherished, loved, and enjoyed. You understand her distress.

## What is the working diagnosis or differential diagnosis?

The child has swallowed a foreign body.

## What do I need to know?

- What is it?
- Where is it?
- Are there any complications?

## Which imaging modality will *confirm*, exclude, define, or show the progress of this?

1. *A sharp or poisonous object*—it must be found. Start with an abdominal film. If negative, proceed to a PA and a lateral of the chest. If negative, proceed to a lateral of the soft tissues of the neck.

2. *Blunt objects*—don't often cause trouble if they reach the abdomen. Start with a PA chest X-ray. If negative, proceed to a lateral of the chest and neck. May need a contrast swallow if radiolucent.

3. *Bones*—fish bones cause so many false-positives and false-negatives that it may be better to treat without X-rays. A lateral of the soft tissues of the neck is a useful image for meat bones.

## What may be shown, and where do I go from here?

### *What if it is normal?:*

- Discuss with the radiographer if another, or a more penetrated, view is needed.
- with a sharp object, ask someone else to check the films;

- with blunt objects and bones treat appropriate to the symptoms or proceed to endoscopy.

*What if it is abnormal?*

- The object is visible.
- Shows a perforation with gas in the soft tissues of the neck or mediastinum or a pneumoperitoneum.
- A swelling of the prevertebral soft tissues of the neck due to an abscess or haematoma.

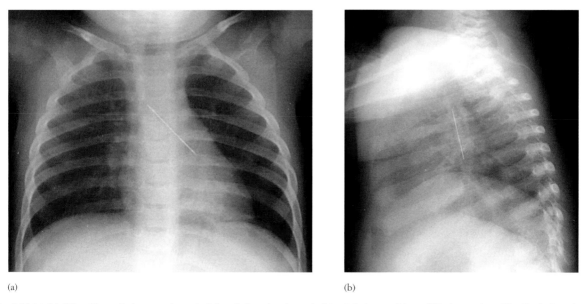

(a)                                                                                     (b)

**Figs 8.10** (a), (b)  Why this needle has gone down the left main bronchus instead of the right is one of those difficult questions. Usually the bronchus intermedius attracts inhaled foreign bodies like a magnet, so that pneumonia at the right base in a child should raise appropriate questions if it does not resolve. The films provide a great lesson in anatomy. The carina, as seen on the lateral film, is more superior than is commonly thought.

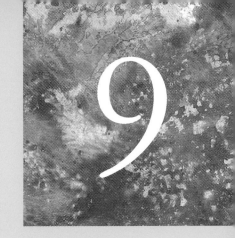

# 9

# *Investigation of the genitourinary system*

- Cases 1–4:

  What is the working diagnosis or differential diagnosis?

  What do I need to know?

  Which imaging modality will confirm, exclude, define, or show the progress of this?

  What may be shown, and where do I go from here?

# Investigation of the genitourinary system

## Case 1

> A 60-year-old man presents with a history of severe, right-sided, colicky, abdominal pain which has been present for 12 hours.
> Urinalysis reveals microscopic haematuria.

### What is the working diagnosis or differential diagnosis?

Ureteric colic, this is often called renal colic.

Cholelithiasis/cholecystitis, GI obstruction, and a leaking abdominal aortic aneurysm need to be considered.

### What do I need to know?

The site and cause of obstruction of the right urinary tract

### Which imaging modality will *confirm*, exclude, define, or show the progress of this?

- Intravenous urogram (IVU)
- CT scan

A CT scan has replaced an IVU in many centres because it:

- is quick (takes 10 minutes);
- detects almost all calculi;
- visualizes dilatation of the collecting system, swelling of the kidney, and perirenal fluid (stranding) which occur with obstruction;
- requires no contrast, either oral or intravenous;
- detects other pathology such as a leaking aortic aneurysm, small bowel obstruction, pneumoperitoneum, pancreatitis, appendicitis, torsion of an ovary, and may show signs of acute cholecystitis

### What may be shown, and where do I go from here?

*What if it is normal?*

- Microscopic haematuria as a finding has raised one of those mental red flags. Investigation must proceed.

## What if it is abnormal?

- An obstruction—since the ureter is a hollow organ an obstruction can be:
  - *luminal*: calculus, blood clot;
  - *mural*: stricture, transitional cell carcinoma;
  - *extramural*: compression by a tumour (carcinoma of the cervix or rectum).

# Intravenous urogram, also called an intravenous pyelogram (IVP)

## Description:

- 50–100 ml of contrast is injected intravenously. A molecule of the contrast contains iodine (often 3 atoms) and has a molecular weight of around 800. Glomeruli allow molecules of this size to be freely filtered. It is not reabsorbed or secreted by the collecting tubules. It does, however, become more concentrated because water is reabsorbed. The contrast fills the nephrons to give a nephrogram and later passes into the pelvicalyceal systems, ureters, and bladder to complete the urogram.

## Preparation:

- A bowel prep. is sometimes useful; fluids are better not restricted.

## Advantages:

- Some clinicians feel comfortable seeing the whole urinary tract on a single film.

## Disadvantages:

- You may need to wait up to 24 hours for the contrast to show the site of obstruction.

## Contraindications:

- If there has been a previous reaction to IV contrast.
- Renal failure
- Pregnancy

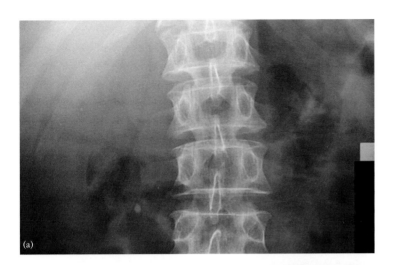

(a)

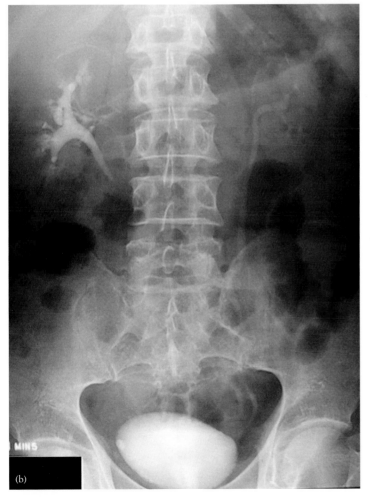

(b)

**Figs 9.1** (a) Preliminary film, (b) IVU at 60 minutes On the right side is an obstruction of the ureter. at the level of the L3–4 intervertebral disc. It is a high-grade obstruction and the cause was shown on a plain film to be a ureteric calculus. Because the glomerular filtrate continues to be generated at up to arteriolar pressure, there is continued accumulation of fluid, which gives dilatation of the pelvicalyceal system and ureter. The contrast is delayed in the collecting tubules. The human body has great homeostatic mechanisms. Some of the pressure in the kidney is relieved by flow of the filtrate into the lymphatic system, called pyelolymphatic backflow and is seen here. Pain is caused by stretching the collecting system and the renal capsule. The left side shows a normal variant, a duplex collecting system. The path of the ureter can be followed to serve as a guide for when one looks for calculi in a plain abdominal X-ray. It descends near the tips of the transverse processes, overlies the sacroiliac joint, and then heads towards the ischial spine before turning medially towards the bladder and site of the ureteric orifice. A phlebolith is visible in the pelvis.

**Fig. 9.2** This non-contrast CT of a 62-year-old man shows the cause of his left loin pain, a calculus at the pelviureteric junction. A staghorn calculus occupies the calyces of the lower pole of the kidney. Dilatation of the collecting system was seen on slices at other levels, indicating obstruction. The other pathology is a small right kidney, probably with diminished function. If the relative function of each kidney needs to be determined, a nuclear imaging study will provide the figures. CT gives good images in the abdomen in people with considerable fat in the mesentery and omentum such as this. Ultrasound is better in thin people.

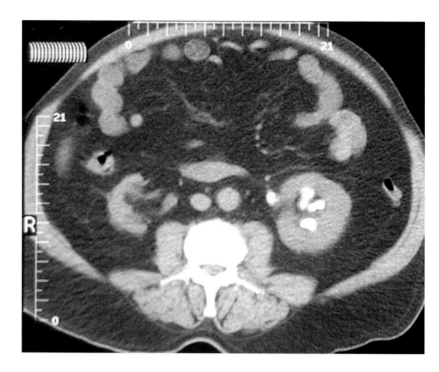

# Case 2

A 40-year-old woman comes to see you with a history of painless, macroscopic haematuria.
Examination is unremarkable.

## What is the working diagnosis or differential diagnosis?

Haematuria for investigation

## What do I need to know?

What is the cause of the bleeding?

## Which imaging modality will confirm, exclude, *define*, or show the progress of this?

Ultrasound of the kidney and abdominal X-ray (AXR) or IVU

# Ultrasound

### Description and uses:

- Bouncing sound waves off the components of the kidney. It shows the morphology of the kidney, the outline as well as the internal structure. The cortex and medulla together constitute the parenchyma and are well demonstrated. Blood flow is perceived when the Doppler capability is used. One sees the pelvicalyceal system and the ureter only when they are dilated.

### Patient preparation:

- nil

### Advantages:

- A relatively quick and cheap examination.
- No radiation is involved.

### Disadvantages:

- Finer detail of the collecting system requires an IVU or, in somebody with impaired renal function, a retrograde pyelogram.

### Contraindications:

- nil

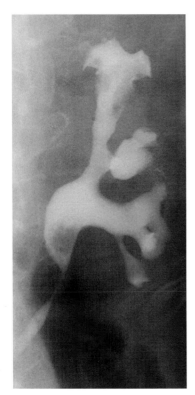

**Fig. 9.4** If the tumour is not in the parenchyma of the kidney, it may be missed on the ultrasound scan. When renal function is impaired, perhaps an IVU cannot be performed or may not show the collecting system with enough clarity for diagnosis. In this situation, a retrograde pyelogram can fill the need for imaging of the pelvicalyceal system and ureter. It is performed by injecting contrast via a ureteric catheter that is inserted following a cystoscopy. Biopsies, brushings, and washings would have been taken at the same time to look for malignant cells in the bladder and ureters. The pyelogram demonstrates a filling defect in the renal pelvis. A second tumour distorts the superior calyx. Transitional cell carcinomas are thought to be caused by urothelial toxins affecting the transitional epithelium and can therefore be multifocal.

## What may be shown, and where do I go from here?
### What if it is normal?

- This is a red flag symptom. Further investigation is mandatory:
  - cystoscopy to check the bladder mucosa and ureters;
  - IVU to look for a transitional cell carcinoma;
  - retrograde pyelogram if the clarity of the IVU images is unsatisfactory or a degree of renal failure excludes the use of an IVU;
  - a CT may be needed to find small renal masses.

### What if it is abnormal?

- A renal mass may be shown, indicating a renal cell carcinoma. The examination could also show if the tumour has entered the renal vein and IVC. Renal cell carcinomas and hepatocellular carcinomas have the characteristic of spreading along venous pathways. Further investigation with CT or MRI would be necessary to assess local spread, determine if the para-aortic nodes were involved, and to check the other kidney. Add a CXR to look for metastases in the lungs.

- The AXR can show urinary tract calcification.

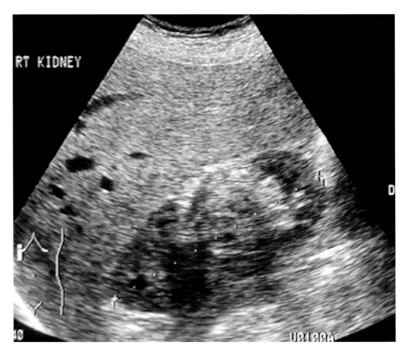

**Fig. 9.3** Ultrasound images do not have the resolution of X-rays but contain information that is not available elsewhere. Look more at the big picture rather than the minutiae of the image. It is not easy to present all the information of the examination on the hard copy. The parenchyma of the kidney is of low echogenicity so it appears dark, darker than the liver. The cursor measures the length of the kidney as 10 cm. In the lower moiety of the kidney is an echogenic mass, about 5 cm in diameter. It is a renal cell carcinoma. Why is it called a carcinoma? Carcinomas are malignant tumours of epithelial cells. This is a cancer of the lining cells of the nephron.

## Case 3

A 20-year-old man comes to see you to seek your advice about a painless swelling of the left side of the scrotum, which he has noticed over the last week. The examination confirms the presence of a lump; it seems to be an enlarged testis. It is not transilluminable. A hydrocoele is unlikely.

## What is the working diagnosis or differential diagnosis?

Testicular neoplasm

## What do I need to know?

- Is the lesion intra- or extratesticular?
- Is it cystic or solid?

## Which imaging modality will confirm, exclude, *define*, or show the progress of this?

Ultrasound

## Ultrasound of the scrotum

### Description and uses:

This is a rapid and not expensive method of examining the scrotal contents for:
- testicular masses and inflammation;
- fluid in the tunica vaginalis;
- epididymitis;
- varicocoele.

### Advantages:

- No other imaging of small parts shows the anatomy and perfusion as well as ultrasound.

### Disadvantages:

- It is not 100% reliable in confirming or excluding testicular torsion, even with sensitive colour Doppler that detects perfusion.

### Patient preparation:

- nil

### Contraindications:

- nil

---

### *Hint*

**Scrotal swelling**

Scrotal swellings are best considered under the classification of:

| | |
|---|---|
| acute painful | testicular torsion, epidiymo-orchitis |
| acute painless | hydrocoele |
| chronic painful | epididymitis |
| chronic painless | tumour: germ cell, or non-germ cell |

### What may be shown, and where do I go from here?

*What if it is normal?*

- The lump must have resolved by the time the examination was performed and probably was inflammatory.

*What if it is abnormal?*

- Testicular tumour
  - germ cell: seminoma or non-seminoma
  - supporting cell: Sertoli cell or Leydig cell

  will need CT to see if the lungs and the mediastinal and abdominal nodes are involved prior to surgery.

- Haematocoele—may need drainage.

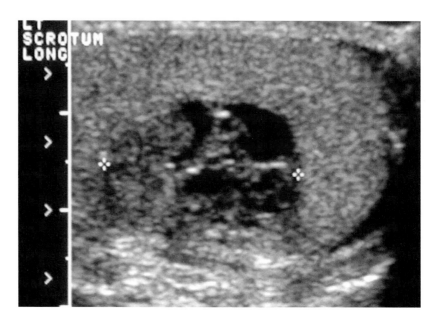

**Fig. 9.5** This is an ultrasound of a man aged 30. Longitudinal image of the left testis. The texture of the testis is usually homogenous. In this scan there is one region of low echogenicity (looks dark/blacker) measuring up to 2 cm in diameter. The appearances are those of a testicular tumour.

# Case 4

A 25-year-old woman comes to see you about vaginal bleeding and some central hypogastric pain. Last normal menstrual period was 7 weeks previously. The examination showed a closed cervix.

A pregnancy test is positive.

## What is the working diagnosis or differential diagnosis?

Threatened abortion
Missed abortion

## What do I need to know?

Is there a live, intrauterine fetus?

## Which imaging modality will *confirm*, exclude, define, or show the progress of this?

Ultrasound, a transvaginal or transabdominal scan

## What may be shown, and where do I go from here?

### What if it is normal?

That means one of two findings

a: normal (empty) uterus, both ovaries identified and looking normal, no abnormal adnexal mass, no free fluid. Could be wrong dates or a complete abortion. Repeat serum bHCG level and ultrasound if indicated. Normally the gestational sac is visible at the fifth week of amenorrhoea, the fetus is detectable at the sixth week, and the heartbeat is seen at 7 weeks. The gestational age is counted from the first day of the last menstrual period. May still need a laparoscopy to exclude ectopic pregnancy and appendicitis.

b: live intrauterine pregnancy (threatened abortion): use expectant management.

### What if it is abnormal?

• Empty sac: it could be a blighted ovum (missed abortion) or early viable pregnancy. Repeat bHCG and ultrasound if indicated.

• Non-viable pregnancy: treat.

• Ectopic pregnancy: treat.

• Indeterminate: a serum bHCG greater than 6,500 mIU/ml and an empty uterus should be considered as an ectopic pregnancy until proven otherwise.

## Transvaginal or transabdominal ultrasound

### Description and uses:

- The transvaginal probe is enclosed in a condom and inserted into the vagina, usually by the patient herself. Information obtained includes the site and number of fetuses, the size of the fetus and calculated period of gestation, and whether it is an ectopic pregnancy.

### Patient preparation:

- The technique requires an empty bladder for a transvaginal examination; a full bladder for a transabdominal examination. It displaces the small bowel loops from the pelvis.

### Advantages:

- Transvaginal examination gives better resolution because the probe is closer to the uterus and a higher frequency is used (5 MHz as against 3 MHz). Some women say it is more comfortable than having a distended bladder.

### Disadvantages:

- It may be difficult to see all of the adnexae.

### Precautions:

- A TV ultrasound needs informed consent. Actually, every examination does, but in this instance it may be better in writing.

**Fig. 9.6** Transabdominal scan. Longitudinal section of the pelvis. The convention is that the cephalad end is to your left. Anterior is the bladder with no echoes in the lumen and therefore appearing black. The uterus has a clearly defined central echo (midline stripe of the endometrium) in the fundus. A distorted gestational sac lies in the lower uterus and extends as low as the cervix. No fetal pole is seen. The vagina is visible, the mucosa giving an echogenic midline stripe. The appearances are of an inevitable abortion.

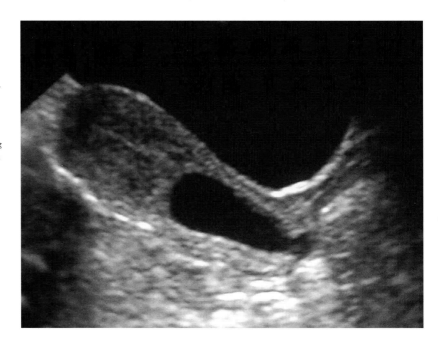

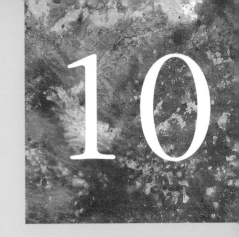

# 10

# Investigation of the musculoskeletal system

- Cases 1–3:

  What is the working diagnosis or differential diagnosis?

  What do I need to know?

  Which imaging modality will confirm, exclude, define, or show the progress of this?

  What may be shown, and where do I go from here?

# Case 1

A 40-year-old male presents with a history of acute onset of low back pain that came on when he stepped out of his car. Further inquiry reveals that the pain radiates down the right leg to the little toe. Examination demonstrates a gait disturbance, loss of the ankle jerk, and weakness of the plantar–flexors of the foot.

It is said that 90% of clinical information is contained in the history. This is a good example. The story is one of an acute soft-tissue injury, low back pain and sciatica, probably from a prolapsed disc. The history is not that of infection, tumour, or an inflammatory disease such as ankylosing spondylitis.

If the clinical problem were acute back pain, ± sciatica, no imaging would be necessary, unless the condition failed to respond to 6 weeks of conservative therapy. The back pain that requires immediate imaging is that with significant sphincter or motor disturbance, or with indicators of neoplasm or infection, or following trauma.

## What is the working diagnosis or differential diagnosis?

Protrusion of the L5–S1 intervertebral disc. Degeneration of the annulus fibrosus has allowed part of the nucleus pulposus to escape into the spinal canal postero-laterally on the right, compressing the S1 nerve root.

## What do I need to know?

The level of the pathology if surgery is the treatment of choice.

## Which imaging modality will confirm, exclude, *define*, or show the progress of this?

MRI. CT, a CT myelogram, or a lumbar myelogram will all be equal to the task, but with different morbidity and cost. The preferred modality depends on local factors such as availability, cost, and preference of the orthopaedic surgeon.

## What may be shown, and where do I go from here?

### *What if it is normal?*

- No neural compression: consider some lesion outside the region of the images.

### What if it is abnormal?

- Neural compression of either the nerve root or thecal sac: seek a surgical opinion.

## MRI of the spinal canal

### Description and uses:

- T1 weighted scans show fluid such as CSF and flowing blood as black. Areas of pathology are usually grey/black on T1 because of the extra cells and oedema. Fat is high signal (white). Anatomical detail is good.
- T2 weighted scans give good imaging of pathology because fluid shows as high signal (white).

### Patient preparation:

- Check for ferromagnetic implants and claustrophobia.

### Advantages:

- Gives excellent soft-tissue contrast.
- The adjacent bone in the vertebrae and pelvis do not give artefacts as can occur with CT.
- Multiplanar imaging is possible.
- No ionizing radiation involved.

### Disadvantages:

- Cost
- Lack of fine bone detail

### Contraindications:

- The presence of ferromagnetic implants

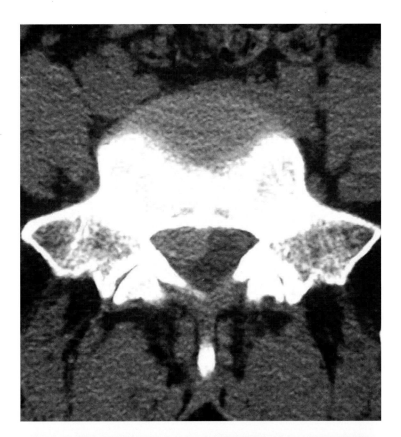

**Fig.** 10.1 CT scan. The L5–S1 level is shown here. Anteriorly, part of the intervertebral disc is imaged obliquely. The dense, cortical bone of the vertebral end plate appears white. The medullary bone of the transverse processes shows its trabecular pattern. A fissure in the annulus fibrosus of the intervertebral disc has allowed part of the nucleus pulposus to herniate into the spinal canal on the right side (of the patient). This disc fragment is of higher attenuation (whiter) than the thecal sac and its contents of CSF and nerve roots. The spinal cord has terminated above at the L1 level. The thecal sac and the nerve roots it contains (S2-S5) have been pushed to the left. The S1 nerve root, which has left the thecal sac on the right side, cannot be seen but it must be irritated

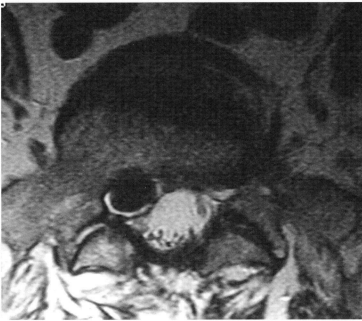

**Fig.** 10.2 A different patient. MRI has the advantage of imaging in any plane. This is one slice of the axial series. The CSF is white, so this is a T2-weighted image (T2WI). The thecal sac and the contained nerve roots are displaced to the left by the disc fragment.

## Case 2

A father brings his 6-year-old son to see you with a history of a limp that has been present for 5 days. Actually, the diagnosis was in your mind from the time the child walked in the door, limping and favouring the left leg. Perthes' disease needs to be excluded.

The rest of the history and examination was directed to evaluating other causes, developing a rapport with the boy and his father and gaining some insight into the social situation. The limp could be a result of any problem from the low back down to the toes. Trauma, infection, and a foreign body were considered and excluded.

## What is the working diagnosis or differential diagnosis?

Perthes' disease of the femoral head

## What do I need to know?

Is there any abnormality of the hip?

## Which imaging modality will *confirm*, exclude, define, or show the progress of this?

Pelvis and left hip X-ray

## What may be shown, and where do I go from here?

### What if it is normal?

- Significant disease is not excluded. It may be in the early phase. Seek an orthopaedic opinion.

### What if it is abnormal?

- Perthes' disease will need specialist treatment.
- In an older child (10–15 years of age), a slipped capital femoral epiphysis could be the cause.

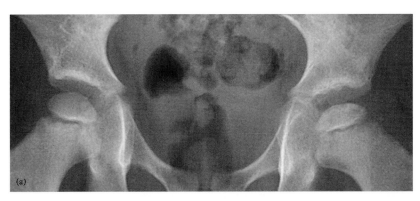

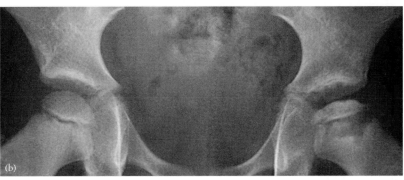

Figs 10.3 (a), (b) The proximal epiphysis of the left femur is initially sclerotic and smaller than that on the right in this 6-year-old boy. Ten weeks later, collapse of the head of the femur and of the superior metaphysis occurs. It looks as if part of the head of the femur dies (osteonecrosis) and that is what it is. It has the name of Perthes' disease. The cause, though, is not clear, probably avascular necrosis from some reason.

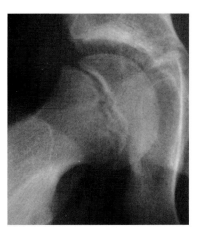

Fig. 10.4 The femur is externally rotated to give a lateral projection. Following the line of the cortex of the neck of the femur reveals a step across the epiphyseal plate, down to the epiphysis that is the head of the femur. This cause of a limp in the early teenage years is appropriately called a slipped capital femoral epiphysis (SCFE).

## Case 3

The 60-year-old former waterfront worker is looking worried. He had gastric carcinoma diagnosed 10 months ago, treated by gastrectomy. A few complications had slowed him down, but he had then started to enjoy what was left of perhaps a short life. You knew the trigger words and had his trust so that he would confide in you his deepest thoughts. It sounded as if he had been reading Tolstoy when he said, 'fear of dying without ever having known love is greater than the fear of death itself. It's not so much death that I am afraid of; more that I will die with my dreams unfulfilled'. His most endearing feature was his love of his family and a regret that he could have spent more time with them. Now he has more time. The illness has cleared his mind so that he can see what is and what isn't important. Today's consultation is to talk about how things are going and to report a couple of worrying symptoms, weight loss and pain in the left ribs.

## What is the working diagnosis or differential diagnosis?

Carcinoma of the stomach

## What do I need to know?

Are there rib secondaries?

Which imaging modality will confirm, exclude, *define*, or show the progress of this?

CXR
Radionuclear bone scan

## Nuclear imaging (footnote 19)

*Bone scan*

*Patient preparation:*

- Ensure hydration.
- No barium studies performed for 1 week prior to the examination. Residual barium absorbs photons.

*Advantages:*

- A radionuclear bone scan is a sensitive test for secondary deposits, stress fractures, and osteomyelitis.

*Disadvantages:*

- Cost

*Contraindications:*

- Caution with pregnancy and breast-feeding

What may be shown, and where do I go from here?

*What if it is normal?*

- It will be a few days later when the result is back. It will be useful to listen to the chest again.

*What if it is abnormal?*

- Multiple 'hot spots' indicating metastases.
- If the areas of increased activity are adjacent to each other in the ribs, they could indicate fractures from a fall that he may not have recalled.

---

19  Also called scintigraphy, nuclear medicine, radionuclear scan (RNS).

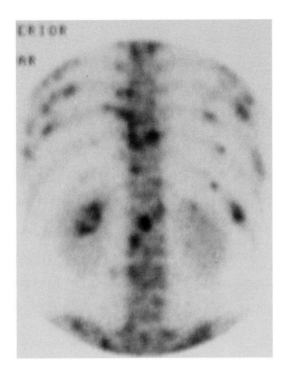

**Fig. 10.5** The increased bone turnover of these metastatic deposits attracts the radiopharmaceutical (technetium attached to MDP) and shows as increased activity. Multiple sites of these deposits are in the ribs, vertebral column, and pelvis—places where there is red marrow in the bone and with a greater blood supply, hence likely targets for metastases.

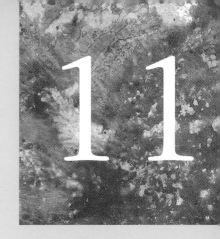

# 11

# Investigation of the central nervous system

- Cases 1–3:

  What is the working diagnosis or differential diagnosis?

  What do I need to know?

  Which imaging modality will confirm, exclude, define, or show the progress of this?

  What may be shown, and where do I go from here?

# Investigation of the central nervous system

## Case 1

> A 40-year-old woman presents with a history of acute onset of a frontal headache, accompanied by vomiting.

### What is the working diagnosis or differential diagnosis?

Subarachnoid haemorrhage

### What do I need to know?

Presence, extent, and complications

### Which imaging modality will *confirm*, exclude, define, or show the progress of this?

CT head scan

## CT head scan

### Description and uses:

- CT has undergone many technical improvements since its origin in 1972. Spiral scanners can now perform a head scan in 15 minutes in an ambulatory patient, with pre- and postcontrast scans. The scan itself can take as little as 10 seconds, and can therefore be performed on some children without the need of a general anaesthetic—it's over before they know it.

### Patient preparation:

- nil

### Advantages:

- It is useful in detecting blood from trauma, hypertensive haemorrhage, or subarachnoid haemorrhage (it detects 90% of acute, non-traumatic SAH). It will show a cerebral infarct after 12 hours and demonstrates primary and secondary tumours and their surrounding oedema.

### Disadvantages:

- Side-effects are a small dose of radiation to the sensitive structure of the lens of the eyes.

## CT head scan (continued)

- Care has to be taken that vomiting with aspiration does not occur with sick people in the supine position who have been injected with the mildly emetic contrast.

### Contraindications:

- Allergy to contrast media would mean that intravenous contrast could not be used.

## What may be shown, and where do I go from here?

### What if it is normal?

- A normal study indicates one of two things: the provisional diagnosis is wrong or the haemorrhage is too small to be detected by CT. This is another way of saying that the sensitivity of CT for detecting SAH is not 100%.

### What if it is abnormal?

- Haemorrhage; high attenuation material in the subarachnoid space and perhaps in the ventricles and brain substance. A contrast study may show the aneurysm or another cause of bleeding.
- A diagnosis that was not suspected may be seen:
  - encephalitis with oedema of the cerebrum, typically of the temporal lobe with herpes encephalitis;
  - ventriculomegaly indicating hydrocephalus of either the obstructive or non-obstructive type;
  - cerebral abscess.

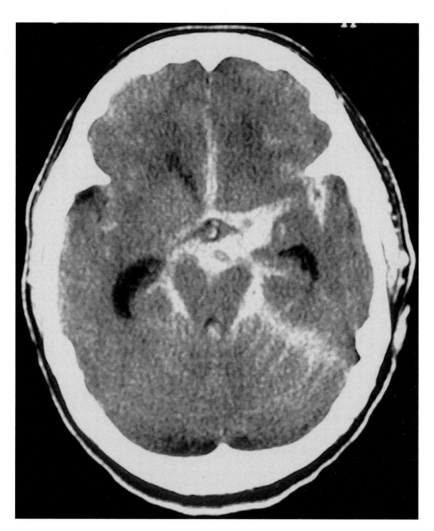

**Fig. 11.1** High-attenuation material is present. It must be blood and it fills the interhemispheric fissure anteriorly, the left middle cerebral (Sylvian) fissure, and the basal cisterns, the interpeduncular in the midline and the ambient, which is lateral to the cerebral peduncles. These cisterns are defined, but communicating, parts of the subarachnoid space. They fill the incongruities between the skull and the base of the brain, a function of fat in the rest of the body. This subarachnoid haemorrhage also extends over the left cerebellar hemisphere. It mixes with the cerebrospinal fluid and can block the absorption of CSF, leading to hydrocephalus, shown here by dilatation of the inferior horns of the lateral ventricles.

## Case 2

A 47-year-old woman has had a grand mal seizure and is brought to your care centre. She is confused but soon recovers and tells her story of a brain tumour that was treated by radiotherapy last year.

## What is the working diagnosis or differential diagnosis?

Epilepsy secondary to a brain tumour

## What do I need to know?

Is there further growth or any complication of the disease or treatment?

## Which imaging modality will confirm, exclude, define, or show the progress of this?

MRI or CT

## Magnetic resonance imaging

### Patient preparation:

- No preparation is usually necessary unless fasting for a general anaesthetic; mascara can degrade images; discuss claustrophobia.

### Contraindications:

- metallic, ferromagnetic implants

## What may be shown, and where do I go from here?

### What if it is normal?

- Check that you are looking at the correct images.

### What if it is abnormal?

- Significant growth of the tumour will provoke a discussion about what, if anything, can be done.

- Hydrocephalus, as a complication of the tumour, surgery, infection, or radio-therapy.

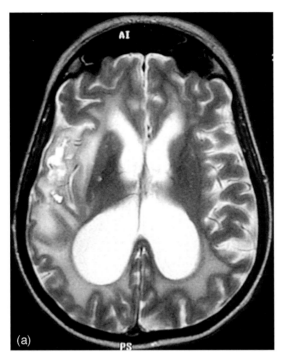 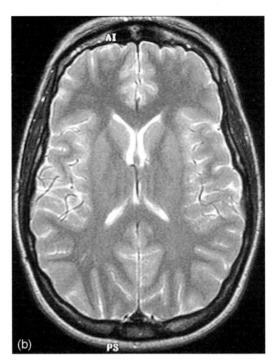

**Figs 11.2** (a), (b)  A normal MRI is also presented here to give some comparison.

How to look at an MRI and not act like a dummy

1.  If using hard copy, find the first film, look for the 'header', the data image at the top left of the sheet, and then place the film correctly oriented on the viewing box.
2.  Determine if it is a T1- or T2-weighted image. T1-weighted images have black CSF. They are useful for clarifying the anatomy. Amateurs should proceed directly to the T2-weighted images that will have white (bright) CSF. Most pathology has oedema, and oedema shows up as white areas on T2.
3.  See if contrast such as gadolinium has been injected.
4.  Look *at* the ventricles, cerebral and cerebellar substance, and the skull and facial structures.
5.  Look *for* something too white, comparing one side with the other.
6.  Look *for* something too black.
7.  Look *for* distortion or displacement of a normal structure.

The ventricles are large, as are the sulci. It looks like loss of cerebral substance secondary to radiation therapy. An abnormal, irregularly shaped white area is detected in the right temporal lobe and is the remains of the tumour. The black areas are the bone of the skull, lumen of the vessels, and gas in the frontal sinuses.

## Case 3

Fred is a 74-year-old man who has been having episodes of weakness in his left arm over the last month. He started smoking at the age of 15 but quit 2 years ago. His BP is 160/96. The only other significant finding on examination was a bruit over the right carotid bifurcation.

### What is the working diagnosis or differential diagnosis?

Transient ischaemic attacks

### What do I need to know?

- Is there any obstruction to blood flow between the heart and the head?
- Is there a site of origin of small emboli?

Examination has targeted the carotid vessels at the bifurcation. They are also implicated epidemiologically as the usual suspects.

### Which imaging modality will *confirm*, exclude, define, or show the progress of this?

Duplex ultrasound of the carotid arteries. Angiography and magnetic resonance angiography (MRA) are alternatives.

## Duplex ultrasound of the carotid arteries

### Description and uses:

- The duplex study, meaning grey-scale imaging and Doppler measurement of flow, assesses intimal thickening, atherosclerotic plaque, and estimates the degree of stenosis by calculating velocity. Studies have shown that increased velocity correlates with certain degrees of stenosis.

### Patient preparation:

- nil

### Advantages:

- non-invasive; no radiation

### Disadvantages:

- It does not demonstrate the plaque with the clarity of angiography but the decision to operate may not require this information.

### Contraindications:

- nil

## What may be shown, and where do I go from here?

### What if it is normal?

- Look for another site of emboli. Check the chest X-ray, and if the heart is suspected of throwing off the emboli order an echocardiogram.

### What if it is abnormal?

- Varying degrees of stenosis. The treatment, medical or surgical, varies with the state of the other arteries supplying blood to the head, symptoms, and general health. A CT head scan will show old or recent areas of brain ischaemia.

- Indeterminate. A technically difficult study or one which provides insufficient information for action to be taken. May need a carotid angiogram.

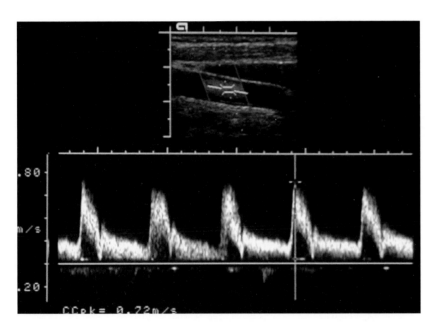

**Fig. 11.3** Images of a carotid duplex study seem to be busy, technical information lining the margins. Only the essentials are shown here. Peak velocity in the common carotid is around 0.72 m/s and it drops to 0.20 m/s at the end of diastole. These are normal flow rates. No sign of intimal thickening or plaque here. The stenosis was more distal.

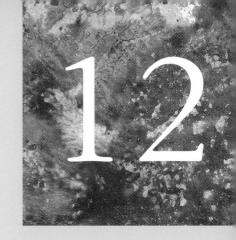

**12**

# Investigation of breast disease

- Cases 1 and 2:
  What is the working diagnosis or differential diagnosis?
  What do I need to know?
  Which imaging modality will confirm, exclude, define, or show the progress of this?
  What may be shown, and where do I go from here?

# Investigation of breast disease

There are many types of breast disease. Radiology is mainly concerned with cancer. In that regard, two scenarios interest us: a woman with, and a woman without, a breast lump.

## Rules

- A screening mammogram every 2 years is useful in an asymptomatic woman, without a breast lump, who is between 50 and 70 years of age.
- Breast lumps need to be treated by specialists.

## Case 1  Screening mammogram

A 55-year-old woman sees you about something, which you diagnose as plantar fasciitis. Her last mammogram was 3 years ago and, at your suggestion, she agrees to have another.

## What is the working diagnosis or differential diagnosis?

Screening mammogram on a well woman

## What do I need to know?

Is the breast tissue normal?

## Which imaging modality will *confirm*, exclude, define, or show the progress of this?

Mammogram

## Mammogram

*Description and uses:*

- The breast is compressed so that a uniform exposure is obtained. An oblique view allows visualization of the axillary tail and a craniocaudal view is taken for additional information. These views are not at right angles.

*Patient preparation:*

- Explain what is to happen and why.

*Advantages:*

- Detects cancers earlier than by palpation and gives an increase in longevity.

## Mammogram (continued)

### Disadvantages:

- Only has a sensitivity of 80%; one in five cancers will not be seen.

### Contraindications:

- nil

## What may be shown, and where do I go from here?

### What if it is normal?

- Most studies will be normal and can be repeated in 2 or 3 years.

### What if it is abnormal?

- Cancers are seen as soft-tissue masses, as irregular and branching micro-calcification in the ducts, or as a distortion of the normal structure.

Fewer than 5 women in every 1000 screened will have breast cancer. Approximately 50 of the 1000 will have an abnormality that requires further assessment such as more radiographs, ultrasound examination, or a fine-needle (23-gauge, cytology) or core (14-gauge, histology) biopsy to either confirm or exclude the presence of cancer. Excision biopsy may be required.

# Case 2

A 40-year-old woman comes to see you because of a breast lump that she has noticed in the inner lower quadrant of her right breast. She has no family history of carcinoma of the breast or other risk factors. Examination reveals a firm, mobile lump and no enlarged nodes.

## What is the working diagnosis or differential diagnosis?

Breast lump for investigation

## What do I need to know?

The name and address of a breast clinic or breast surgeon

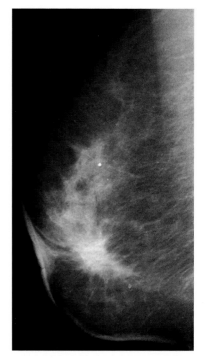

**Fig. 12.1** The parenchyma of the breast, the glandular and stromal elements, are white. One area is more dense (whiter), and contains microcalcification which is difficult to see here. It is causing retraction of the nipple. Two small foci of benign calcification are visible. The black areas that make up most of the breast are adipose tissue. The pectoralis major muscle lies posteriorly. Three features identify carcinoma of the breast—two are opacities and one is distortion of normal structures:

(1)  a mass lesion, poorly defined, and sometimes spiculated (sharp, needle-like projections);

(2)  microcalcification, irregular and branching;

(3)  distortion of the breast tissue, retraction of the nipple or skin.

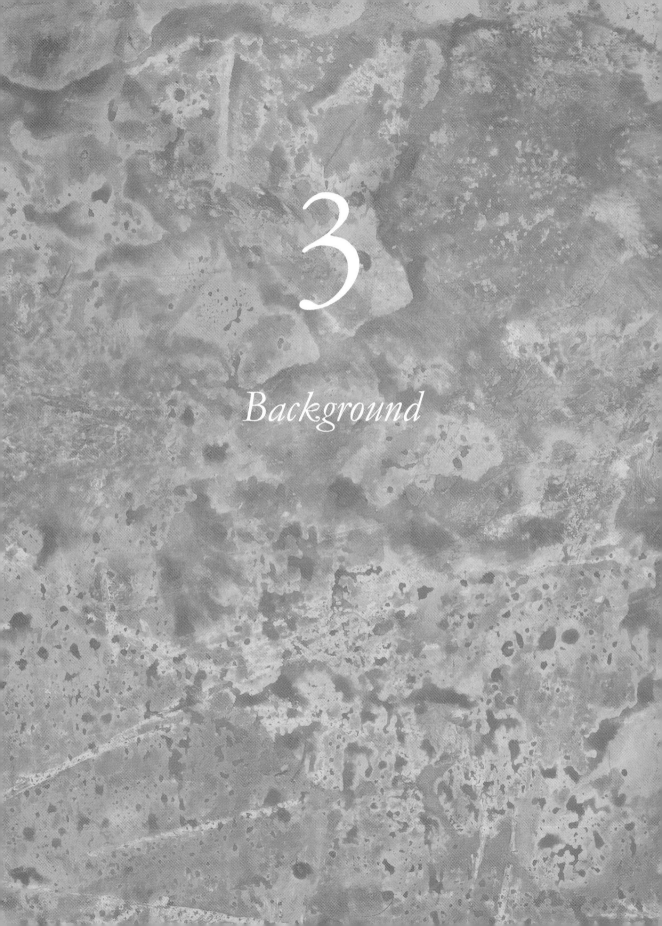

3

*Background*

# Background

The main focus and objectives of this section are to provide important information about:

(1) safety and risk management (Chapter 13):

- contrast media used in medical imaging
- care of the patient
- diagnoses which are easily missed
- radiation minimization (protection)
- policy on X-raying women who may be pregnant;

(2) interventional radiology—a brief guide to some of the available procedures (Chapter 14);

(3) how can radiology help—how to use it for diagnosis, staging disease, planning management, intervention, assessment of treatment, demonstrating any complications, and monitoring for relapse (Chapter 15); and

(4) understanding imaging modalities (Chapter 16).

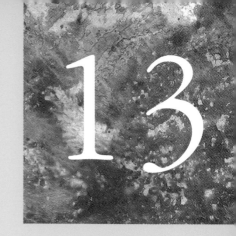

# Safety and risk management

- Contrast media:
  *Types of contrast and uses*
  *Contraindications*
  *Reactions*
  *How to treat reactions*

- Care of the patient:
  *Patient preparation*
  *Ability of ill patients to tolerate investigations*
  *Surveillance after a radiological procedure*
  *Working together with the radiology department*

- Diagnoses which are easily missed

- Radiation minimization (protection)

- Policy on X-raying women who may be pregnant

# Safety and risk management

The first rule of medicine is 'do no harm'. That makes this chapter important. It teaches about safety with respect to medical imaging. The radiologist takes ultimate responsibility for the care of patients in the imaging department. However, fewer adverse events will occur if the clinician flags problem cases so that these people can receive special attention. It is like the added safety measure of having a film read by a radiologist, even though it may have already been assessed in the emergency department and management started on that information. Checks and balances = risk minimization = smart medicine.

What do you need to know?

1. Contrast can cause morbidity and death. It is therefore useful to know which types are available, when to use them, and a little about the reactions they can cause.

2. Care of the patient. How to prepare patients for imaging, assessing whether ill patients will be able to tolerate investigations, what to look for after the procedure, and how to make things easier through cooperation with the radiology practice.

3. Diagnoses which are easily missed (so they won't be). Some important diseases that are uncommon, but serious and treatable, need a little emphasis.

4. Radiation minimization (protection). How to minimize radiation exposure to patients and staff.

5. Policy on X-raying women who may be pregnant. Some guidelines are given.

## Contrast media

(1) Types of contrast and uses

(2) Contraindications

(3) Reactions

(4) How to treat reactions

### Types of contrast and uses

#### Low density

##### Air

Air is introduced into the oesophagus, stomach, and duodenum during a barium swallow and meal to give a double-contrast effect, with the barium coating the mucosa. A similar technique is used with a double-contrast barium enema but $CO_2$ is preferred because it is absorbed quickly, therefore minimizing discomfort. Air is also used for double-contrast arthrograms.

##### $CO_2$

Carbon dioxide is used for barium enemas and occasionally for angiography.

**Fig.** 13.1 Barium can be used as a single-contrast study when it fills the lumen, or as a double-contrast investigation in which case a more concentrated form is used and $CO_2$ or air is added, as shown here. The coating on the mucosa can reveal inflammatory (shown as ulcers) or neoplastic (lumps) disease as well as strictures and diverticula. This barium enema allows visualization of a polyp of the sigmoid colon in the left iliac fossa. Polyp is a generic diagnosis and means tissue arising from the mucosa. Specifically, this is probably an adenoma: tubular, villous, or tubulovillous. Carcinoma can develop, and may already be present, so it should be removed.

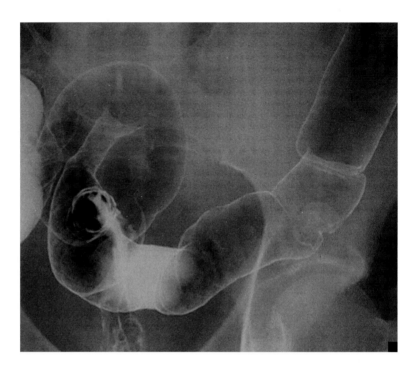

## High density

### Barium

Barium has a high atomic number of 56, which means it has 56 protons and 56 electrons. These cause considerable attenuation of the X-ray beam compared with the soft tissues of the body which comprise mainly carbon (atomic number of 6), hydrogen (atomic number of 1), and oxygen (atomic number of 8). It is only used for demonstrating parts of the gastrointestinal tract. Barium sulfate, an insoluble form of barium, is the appropriate choice and is quite safe except if it escapes from the GIT. Leakage into body cavities may excite a granulomatous inflammatory reaction. Accidental aspiration in small quantities sometimes occurs despite precautions, but causes little harm. Aspiration of larger quantities of barium requires physical therapy to aid removal.

### Water-soluble media

Iodine has an atomic number of 53. It is the essential atom of these important compounds that can be injected intravascularly or into any cavity, sinus, or tract to demonstrate morphology. Sometimes the injection gives an indication of function, for example when it is filtered by the kidney during an IVU. Outline of the kidney and ureter indicates that the kidney is working.

Two major groups of these media have been developed. One is ionic and usually hyperosmolar (700–2100 mOsmol/l, compared to blood which is 265–300 mOsmol/l). The other is a more recent development and is non-ionic, of lower osmolality (300–700 mOsmol/l), safer, and has fewer reactions—but it is more expensive.

Iodine-based media are used in (not all these studies are demonstrated in this book):

- angiograms looking for stenosis, occlusion, site of bleeding, and blood supply;
- venograms to detect thrombosis in the upper limbs when a central venous line is malfunctioning, or in the lower limbs;
- CT examinations to opacify the: systemic arteries; pulmonary arteries for emboli; parenchyma of organs such as the brain, liver, and kidney; veins (portal venous system); urinary tract. Contrast injected intravascularly rapidly becomes distributed in the intravascular and interstitial compartments of the extracellular fluid (ECF), but not in normal brain tissue. Contrast enhancement occurs in the brain when there is a breakdown of the blood–brain barrier, a result of inflammation or of the neovascularization of tumours;
- myelograms when MRI is not available. The contrast is injected into the cerebrospinal fluid (CSF) in the subarachnoid space to look for filling defects: intramedullary, subarachnoid, and extradural;
- cystograms, urethrograms, micturating cystourethrograms and nephrostograms, checking the lines and valves of the urinary tract;
- sinograms and fistulograms to see where the tract leads;
- contrast swallows where there is a risk of aspiration;
- GI studies where there is a chance of perforation/leakage;
- galactograms to find a polyp in a breast duct;
- dacrocystograms to find a site of the block in the tear duct and nasolacrimal duct;
- sialograms of the parotid or submandibular ducts for blocked salivary ducts and the recurrent infection of sialectasis;
- ERCPs, searching for stones, strictures, and neoplasms in the biliary tree; and
- hysterosalpingograms to detect a blockage in the fallopian tubes or other causes of infertility.

## Gadolinium contrast media

These are as useful in MRI as iodine-based contrast is in CT. Gadolinium has a large magnetic moment and works by decreasing the relaxation time.

It is safe. Mortality from injection is around 1 in 1 000 000.

## Fluids with microbubbles

The use of these fluids provides contrast in specialized areas of ultrasound.

## Contraindications of iodine-based contrast

A previous reaction to a contrast injection precludes its subsequent use. Take care with very young, old, pregnant, diabetic, asthmatic, atopic, and dehydrated patients and those with cardiac or renal failure, sickle cell disease, and myeloma.

## Reactions

The mortality rate of these injections is around 1 in 100 000. Mild reactions also occur in the form of nausea, vomiting, and itching. Moderately severe reactions include angioneurotic oedema and dyspnoea. A full explanation of the types of reactions and their treatment must be sought by anyone who has to give one of these injections.

## How to treat reactions

The basic treatment for a severe reaction to IV contrast where there is cardiorespiratory compromise is:

- seek help;
- give oxygen;
- slowly give 1–5 ml of 1 in 10 000 adrenaline (epinephrine), i.e. 0.1–0.5 mg, in cases of bronchospasm or laryngospasm, via the IV line which should still be in place;
- look for and treat hypotension, bradycardia, pulmonary oedema, and cardiac and respiratory arrest appropriately.

## Care of the patient

(1) Patient preparation;

(2) Ability of ill patients to tolerate investigations;

(3) Surveillance after a radiological procedure;

(4) Working together with the radiology department.

## Patient preparation

For a complex radiological procedure, such as placing a stent across an obstruction in the biliary tree, use the following checklist of six items:

1. Review the indications and contraindications.

2. Obtain informed consent.

3. Check the pathology results.

4. Give premedication.

5. Establish an IV line.

6. Cover with antibiotics.

Less complex procedures such as an aortobifemoral angiogram may require only a review of the indications and contraindications, a consent, and an IV line.

## Ability of ill patients to tolerate investigations

When seriously ill people need radiological investigation or management the decision of what to do is complex. It involves consideration of what information is required, what is already available, and which test is suitable. As such, it needs the collaboration of a clinician and an imaging specialist.

Make use of any opportunity to visit the medical imaging centre and see what is involved.

## Surveillance after a radiological procedure

Observe for:

- Bleeding: continue surveillance of the puncture site for 8 hours.

- Bacteraemia and septic shock can accompany or follow interference with an obstructed urinary tract or biliary tree. It should be recognized by hypotension, pallor, and malaise. The pulse can be fast or slow.

- Contrast reactions usually occur in the imaging department. Delayed reactions can present in the form of rashes and itching. Usually no treatment is necessary. The radiologist should be notified and observations continued. The patient is given written information about the name of the contrast material and warned about the possibility of an allergic reaction to any future contrast injections.

- Renal impairment of a mild degree can occur and is more likely in someone who has pre-existing kidney disease.

- If a drain is not working contact whoever put it in. For removal, it is best to contact the radiologist. These drains have cunning locking devices that are only easy to release if you know how. Often a wire is inserted to straighten the tube, allowing easier, less traumatic removal.

## Working together with the radiology department

- *Know what is involved.* Get to know what you are asking your patient to experience.

- *Know what to order.* Specify exactly what you want, for example an X-ray of the forearm, wrist, scaphoid, or hand.

- *If you don't know what to order* tell the radiologist what you want to know and he or she will advise on the best modality.

- *Communication* at formal and informal meetings helps. Call in to see the radiologist. It gets lonely working in a windowless environment.

- *Questioning reports* is healthy and sharpens the minds of both parties.

- *Asking advice* is in the best interests of the patient. Radiologists must be some of the most approachable people in the world.

## Diagnoses which are easily missed

A brief word is appropriate about diagnoses that are delayed and missed because if one is alert for them they won't be.

- *Stress fracture*—the average time from onset of symptoms to diagnosis is 3 months. Presents as pain in the lower leg, ankle, and foot often following increased activity. Diagnosed by a radionuclear scan.

- *Vasculitis*—this is an inflammation of the vessel walls. Can be in the large, medium, or small arteries and presents in such variable ways that it may be some time before the correct diagnosis is considered. In the meantime, batteries of tests, including imaging, are ordered and can be inconclusive. Be alert in a middle-aged person who is unwell with vague pains and aches, abdominal pain, headache, perhaps some renal impairment, and an elevated ESR.

- *Epidural abscess*—presents with back pain and mild fever in a diabetic. Not seen on plain films. Hopefully diagnosed with an MRI before the long tract signs develop.
- *Non-accidental injury in the child at risk*—plain films, radionuclear bone scan, and CT of the head can help with the diagnosis.
- *Osteoid osteoma*—back pain in a young adult, relieved by aspirin. Diagnose with a plain film or nuclear imaging.
- *Psychiatric* disorders—these are sometimes missed because the emphasis is on somatic disease. The clues are in the history, not in the images.

The medical insurance industry still has problems with the failure of clinicians to diagnose:

- fractures of the femur, cervical and thoracic spine, ankle, foot, and scaphoid;
- carcinoma of the breast;
- appendicitis;
- melanoma;
- carcinoma of the cervix; and
- ectopic pregnancy.

## Radiation minimization (protection)

The harmful effects that radiation can produce are divided into two types: those that inhibit cell growth and lead to cell death; and those that modify cell DNA (chromosomes), resulting in cancer, genetic defects, and fetal damage. Particularly sensitive structures are the lenses of the eyes, gonads, lymph nodes, and bone marrow.

Cell death and the inhibition of cell growth are the aims of radiotherapy. It causes these effects by breaking one or both of the DNA strands. The cell will die when it attempts to divide. DNA rupture is caused either by the free radicals produced from the water that makes up 80% of the cell, or directly from the radiation.

Diagnostic radiology operates at much lower doses and power than radiotherapy, around 100 kVp (a peak of 100 000 volts). Radiotherapy uses up to 10 000 000 volts. The problem for diagnostic radiology is not so much of cell death and inhibition of growth, but that theoretically a single photon can displace an electron, create a free radical, and produce cancer or other chromosomal diseases.

Where do ionizing photons come from? (See RCR 1995.) The total ionizing radiation to the average human comes from:

- natural background radiation, mainly from extraterrestrial sources (85%); and
- man-made radiation (15%), of which 97% is from diagnostic radiology.

Up to a quarter of the radiation from diagnostic radiology comes from CT. CXRs are performed much more frequently but have a small dose, 0.03 millisieverts (mSv) for a PA film (20 cm thick adult, 400 speed screen/film system). Interestingly, 0.03 mSv is equivalent to 4 days of natural background radiation or the added cosmic radiation of a 7-hour airline flight such as London to New York (Mohler 1996). A lateral CXR gives five times the dose of a PA film.

Doctors and patients do not think in millisieverts, so to compare various imaging modalities the following table is expressed in PA CXR units. It gives the equivalent risk of different X-ray examinations, having made an allowance for the dose and radiosensitivity of the tissues affected (Enright 1998, personal communication).

Table 13.1
## Risks of ionizing radiation investigations

| Investigation | Risk (effective dose) compared to a PA CXR |
|---|---|
| CXR (PA film) | 1 |
| Lumbar spine (three views) | 100 |
| Abdomen (supine and erect) | 50 |
| IVU | 150 |
| CT head | 100 |
| CT chest | 300 |
| CT abdomen | 400 |
| Radionuclear scan of bone | 200 |

Minimizing radiation dose, particularly to people with chronic diseases, will be beneficial. The protective measures are the responsibility of the radiology clinic or department, but there are several areas where you can help:

- request the use of mobile equipment as little as possible;
- become comfortable reading a PA CXR without a lateral view;
- wear protective clothing;
- order only the minimum number of X-rays.

How to order only the minimum number of X-rays:

1. Follow the thinking pattern described in Section 2 of this book.

2. Use ultrasound or MRI if appropriate.

3. Before ordering an imaging investigation satisfy yourself by answering these questions:

   (a) will the imaging, if either positive or negative, induce a change in the management?—if it won't, don't bother with the test;

   (b) have previous tests been reviewed?

   (c) what is the best modality, considering:

      (i) the cost

      (ii) availability

      (iii) sensitivity and specificity

      (iv) morbidity and mortality of the test?

4. Follow guidelines for the use of radiography such as the Ottawa ankle rules (Verma *et al.* 1997).

5. Some X-rays do not provide significant information that will alter the management or the outcome of the disease, for instance:

   • when there is already enough information to take action or to exclude significant disease;

   • when there is only a remote possibility of the disease being present. Hardison (1979) lists some excuses which have been used to justify further tests: 'to be complete', 'as long as he's in hospital we might as well', 'we're in an academic institution', 'malpractice avoidance', 'it's the protocol', 'if it were my mother I would want it done', and finally 'how do we know he doesn't have it?' to which one replies 'apart from it being a wild guess, with nothing in the history or physical examination to remotely suggest it, we don't'.

6. Radiation exposure to the population will decrease and money will be saved if the following X-rays are ordered sparingly (after Helms 1989):

   • *nasal bones*: leave it for the specialist to order if required;

   • *lateral chest*: ask for it only if you have a problem with the PA film;

   • *skull*: only for a depressed skull fracture or intracranial metal fragments;

   • *sinuses*: only for an unusual presentation or someone who does not respond to treatment;

   • *ribs*: diagnosing a rib fracture does little to change management—a chest X-ray, however, is needed to confirm or exclude a haemopneumothorax;

   • *coccyx*: not only is it difficult to diagnose a fracture here but there is also a large radiation dose to the gonads. Management is not affected. It is difficult to apply a plaster cast, and I have yet to see one internally fixed;

   • *lumbar spine*: no significant radiology finding is usual in acute back strain where there are no neurological signs. X-ray in 6 weeks if symptoms have not resolved with conservative treatment.

Radiologists (and others) recognize that clinical work is not easy. Occasionally the situation arises where at the end of the history and examination the clinician is struggling with unlikely diagnoses. Sometimes an X-ray is ordered. The reason can be to exclude a serious but unlikely illness, to buy time, placing trust in the body's healing powers, or to get a second opinion by asking the patient to return for the results on your day off.

These are the cases where it is important to return to the basics and think: 'What do I need to confirm, exclude, or define?' Make good notes to the radiologist asking for assistance, or better still, telephone or call to see her.

If cases like this are becoming numerous it is time to revise the history-taking technique. Is the problem being identified? Are there psychological or administrative problems when you are trying to diagnose a somatic illness? Finally, is it time to review that brochure in the bottom drawer about continuing medical education?

## Policy on X-raying women who may be pregnant

Policies vary but a few notes may be useful:

1. Find out what the local policy is and follow it.

2. In any person an X-ray may cause some harm and it also uses resources (costs money).

3. The advantage of an X-ray must outweigh the disadvantages.

4. The advantage is increased information.

5. The disadvantages are cost, morbidity and mortality, false-negatives, and false-positives. The morbidity is increased in a woman who is or who may be pregnant. This is particularly applicable in X-rays of the abdomen and pelvis.

6. Use all reasonable methods to determine if the woman is pregnant.

7. In pregnant women delay the X-ray until after the delivery, or use ultrasound or MRI if possible. X-rays in the 10 days from the beginning of a woman's last period are the safest as pregnancy is very unlikely.

8. Organ development is thought to occur from the time of the first missed period and continue for 4 months. As it is primarily organ development that is adversely affected by exposure to radiation, it is during this time that X-rays are to be avoided. Up until the first missed period (the first 2 weeks of fetal development) is not a critical time for damage to organ development.

9. If all else fails refer to the first point.

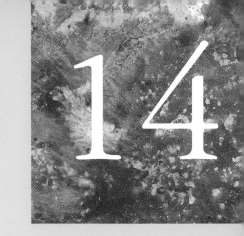

# 14

*Interventional radiology*

# Interventional radiology

Interventional radiology is about using image guidance instead of direct vision to perform therapeutic manoeuvres. It adds treatment to the normal radiology role of diagnosis. The techniques are finding more applications because there is only a small entry wound, usually for a catheter, healing is quicker, and the average length of stay in hospital is shorter.

This chapter teaches how to prepare a patient for an interventional radiological procedure and gives a few examples of these.

If one of your patients is to undergo a complex radiological procedure, follow the checklist below which contains six items:

1. *Review the indications and contraindications.*

2. *Informed consent* should be obtained prior to any procedure. In retrospect, it is never a problem when things go well. But in a surprisingly large number of cases, something happens that is not optimal. In such circumstances, whether a complaint is received from the patient depends to some extent on how the situation was managed, and how the consent was obtained. If the decision to treat is made by the doctor, and the consent is looked on as a side-show on the road to action, there is the potential for trouble. A better scenario is the concept that the decision is made not *with* the patient but *by* the patient at the time of signing the consent. Take time to explain the procedure so that the patient is satisfied that this decision is for the best.

3. *Premedication* is often unnecessary, but a sedative or anxiolytic can be offered to those who would benefit.

4. An *IV line* should be in place to give antibiotics, analgesics, narcotics, fluids, and resuscitation drugs.

5. *Investigations*:

   (a) Coagulation profile. Mandatory if there is liver disease or a history of bleeding. Check if the medications include heparin, warfarin, or aspirin, as these will usually need to be discontinued, sometimes days in advance.

   (b) A knowledge of renal function is useful in those who are to be given large quantities of IV contrast.

   (c) Haemoglobin, electrolytes, and liver function tests are required in patients who are particularly unwell.

6. *Antibiotics* are needed when an obstructed system or abscess is entered or drained.

   Intervention takes many forms including:

- biopsy. A 22-G needle is used for fine-needle aspiration biopsy (FNAB). It has an outside diameter of 0.7 mm and cannot do much harm even if it passes through a vessel or loop of bowel. A drop or two of fluid is obtained. The cytologist prepares an air-dried, Giemsa-stained smear (or similar) and examines the slide for malignant cells. A second pass can obtain material for microbiological analysis.

- core biopsy. Sometimes a well-differentiated tumour requires tissue architecture for diagnosis. A core biopsy can be taken with an 18-G cutting needle (outside diameter of 1.5 mm).

- decompression/drainage of the urinary tract (percutaneous nephrostomy), GIT, or of the biliary tree. Drainage allows the function of the organ to continue, while awaiting the optimal time to attack the cause of the obstruction.

- drainage of abscesses and fluid collections. A catheter can be left in place to drain the collection over several days.

- embolization. This is used to control bleeding or to infarct a tumour.

- angioplasty. Dilates a narrowed artery.

- insertion of stents and IVC filters. Stents are inserted to hold a tubular structure open, perhaps an artery, vein, bile duct, or the oesophagus.

- IVC filters. These block the passage of clots.

- thrombectomy/thrombolysis. Achieved using a potent thrombolytic agent such as urokinase or streptokinase, delivered by a catheter at the site of the thrombus.

- fallopian tube catheterization. This is used to treat some cases of infertility where there is a proximal obstruction of the tube caused by a plug of mucus.

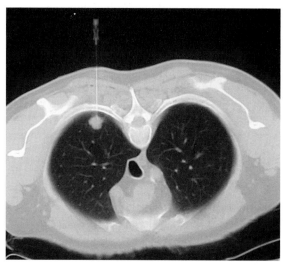

Fig. 14.1 Central lung lesions are often accessible for biopsy at the time of bronchoscopy. Peripheral lesions can be approached percutaneously as long as the patient agrees and there is no bleeding disorder or severe bullous lung disease. This image shows a 22-gauge lumbar puncture needle that is 9 cm long. The tip is in the tumour. A CXR will be performed in 2 hours to exclude a pneumothorax. Seeding of tumour cells along the needle track rarely occurs.

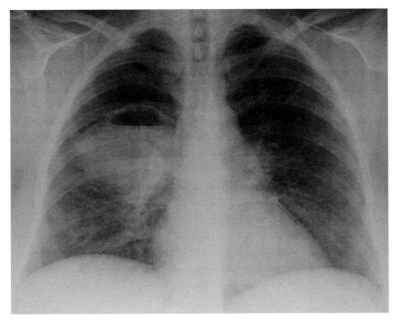

(a)

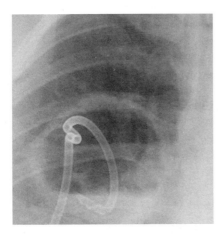

(b)

**Figs 14.2** (a), (b) Drainage of collections can be performed percutaneously. Surgery is also a percutaneous technique, but common usage associates the term with imaging-guidance, insertion of needles, wires, and catheters. This lung abscess extended to the pleura and was easily accessible.

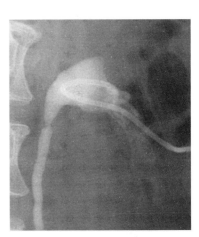

**Fig. 14.3** A nephrostomy tube has been inserted into the left renal pelvis. A loop is formed at the end to discourage accidental dislodgement. Contrast has been injected and it shows a filling defect in the lower calyx, presumably blood clot. The upper ureter is demonstrated. The obstruction is in the distal ureter in the pelvis. The narrowing near the pelviureteric junction is temporary, a peristaltic wave. Nephrostomies allow temporary drainage when there is obstruction, usually by a stone or cancer, and when internal stents cannot be used.

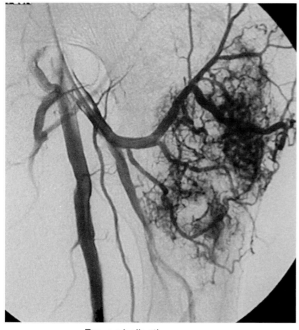
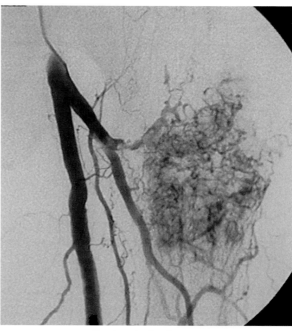

Pre-embolisation                    Post-embolisation

**Figs 14.4** (a), (b) A renal cell carcinoma had caused a pathological fracture of the proximal shaft of the femur. Preoperative embolization was performed to decrease intraoperative bleeding. Small pieces of Gelfoam® were introduced to block the arterial lumen and cause thrombosis.

**Figs 14.5** (a), (b) Atrial fibrillation was the underlying disease and a piece of thrombus embolized to the popliteal artery. The distal end of the filling defect has the smooth shape of an embolus. Collateral circulation preserved the distal perfusion. Treatment was by thrombolysis using a pulsed spray and overnight slow infusion of streptokinase, by the catheter seen here with its tip abutting the clot. The procedure was successful, leaving some small mural thrombi.

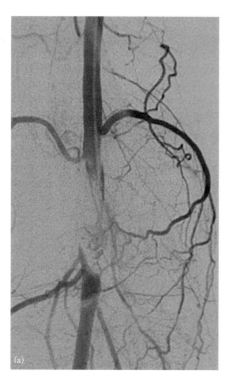
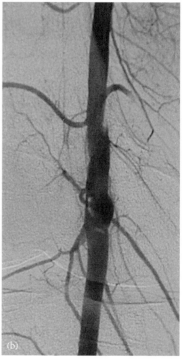

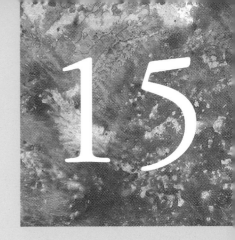

# 15

# How can radiology help

This chapter contains important information

# How can radiology help

## What is radiology about?

The previous chapters have described a system for interpreting radiographs and for the imaging of common clinical problems. It is time to put that information into perspective.

This chapter will explain:

- the role of radiology in providing useful information;
- why imaging is ordered;
- when imaging is ordered;
- typical pathway of clinical thinking processes;
- what variables to consider when ordering investigations;
- what does it mean if the test is normal?
- what does it mean if the test is abnormal?
- how to avoid errors of interpretation;
- how a radiologist can help;
- probabilities.

Finally, it will put radiology in perspective.

## The role of medical imaging

A significant part of medical imaging concerns interventional techniques and these are discussed in Chapter 12. The major role is *providing information*. This information, like vegetables in the corner store, is perishable and its value deteriorates exponentially with time.

*The definition of the role of radiology therefore starts like this*: to provide imaging that gives information to the referring clinician in the shortest time.

## Why imaging is ordered

Because more information is required to:

- *confirm* or *exclude* a diagnosis;
- *define* the anatomy or the extent of the disease, or the functional status;
- follow the *progress of* a disease process.

## When is imaging ordered?

The appropriate *time* for imaging becomes clear when it is put in the proper perspective. To do that we need to look at the *typical pathway of clinical thinking processes*.

## Typical pathway of clinical thinking processes

(1) the history

(2) the provisional diagnosis

(3) the examination

(4) what if there is not enough information as yet

(5) the treatment

(6) ordering another test

## The history

Each of the major diseases, and there are only about 200 of them, should be summarized in one sentence. That pathological definition will:

- be the foundation on which all other information is added;
- explain the symptoms and signs;
- allow other more complex information to be added by association at a later date;
- save time, using cognitive rather than behavioural learning;
- provide a clear, sharp focus which can be remembered for life;
- simplify decision making;
- explain the radiological appearances;
- allow understanding of treatment options.

Look at this one-sentence definition of a complex disease, rheumatoid arthritis, and see if you can guess what will be the symptoms, signs, radiological appearances, and treatment: Rheumatoid arthritis is a chronic, systemic, inflammatory disorder thought to be immunological in origin, which attacks and destroys the joints with a proliferative synovitis and also affects the lungs, heart, blood vessels, muscles, and skin.

A patient arrives with symptoms, and the history is taken. The history taking provides 90% of the clinical information and serves three critical roles:

(1) to identify the problem and determine a provisional diagnosis;

(2) to put the illness in the context of the person's life—what can reasonably be achieved considering the age of the person, prior and concurrent illnesses, effect of the illness, lifestyle and social situation, and the expectations of the patient;

(3) to establish a relationship with the patient, a mutual trust that allows understanding of the diagnosis, treatment, uncertainties, and complications that may occur—part of the recipe for success and your best defence against a lawsuit.

The first question to be answered is: 'Why has this person come to see me at this particular time?' (identifying the problem, what is the hypothesis?). Is it because of:

- some microscopic or macroscopic pathology that I should be able to find?
- pathology that I can deduce is there but cannot be seen, e.g. low back strain?
- functional pathology, e.g. hypertension?
- a behavioural or psychiatric disorder?
- normal development such as pregnancy, or advice? (Confirmation of normality may be a frequent motive for a consultation in primary care.)
- an administrative matter: 'Doc, I've had a week off work. Can you please give me a certificate?'

If the patient is placed in the wrong category, it will lead to frustration and disappointment on both sides.

The history, examination, and investigations are all used to refine or reject the provisional diagnosis (hypothesis).

## Provisional diagnosis

By the end of the history a decision should be made into which category the consultation falls. Classically, students were taught to wait until the *end of the examination* before reaching a provisional diagnosis. The better one becomes at making a diagnosis the earlier it is made, preferably during or at the end of the history taking. Certainly if the diagnosis is made from the history it is the least expensive way to do it. A diagnosis cannot be made if the disease is not understood.

## Examination

The examination can then be likened to the first test or investigation; not an extensive, but a focused study. It will confirm, exclude, define, or demonstrate the progress of a disease. It may be able to confirm the presence of cardiac failure, exclude the presence of retinal vein thrombosis, define the extent of a squamous cell carcinoma in the neck, or assess the progress of a hamstring sprain.

## Not enough information as yet?

How certain is the diagnosis? Is there enough information to take action or exclude significant disease?

Consider the probability of the diagnosis to be somewhere on a line that has a range of 0% to 100%. The line represents the chance of the diagnosis being correct.

### Hint

The making of a diagnosis can take one of two paths:

(1) leaving the decision about the diagnosis until all the information is in. A recipe for expensive and confused medicine with many tests and consequent false-positives and false-negatives.

(2) continuous assessment and upgrading of the data from the history and, if needed, from the examination and tests. The aim is to make an early decision about the provisional diagnosis and acquire just enough information from the history, examination, and tests to pass the action or exclusion threshold and commence treatment. Leads to quicker decisions.

### Hint

Learning in the medical course can take three tracks:

(1) soaking up all knowledge indiscriminately and trying to learn everything (this turns out a confused thinker who has difficulty making decisions, but who thinks his or her knowledge is adequate and who has spent too much time studying and not enjoying it);

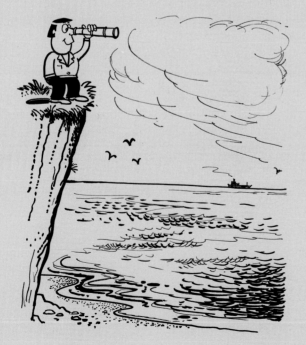

**Fig. 15.1** Learning the medical course No. 1.

## Hint (continued)

(2) drawing a line around a body of knowledge and saying this has to be known, learning is often by memory and repetition (suboptimal technique);

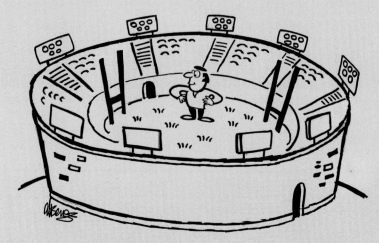

**Fig. 15.2** Learning the medical course No. 2.

(3) using the one-sentence definition of diseases as a base on which other knowledge is added by association (preferred option)—favours minimization of effort and complexity.

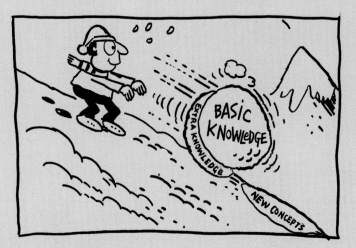

**Fig. 15.3** Learning the medical course No. 3.

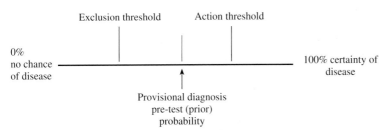

**Fig.** 15.4 Probability of disease.

The action threshold will be close to 100% for diseases like cancer because the treatment is dangerous. Whereas for pharyngitis you may be comfortable to start treatment with penicillin tablets when you are only 80% sure of the diagnosis.

The aim of the clinician is to move the probability of the disease above the action threshold so that treatment can commence, or to move the probability of a serious disease below the exclusion threshold. The probability is moved by information acquired. Often at the end of the examination, and sometimes even at the end of the history, the action threshold has been passed and treatment can commence. If neither the action nor the exclusion threshold has been exceeded, more information is needed. Call for radiology or pathology.

The answer to the question: 'When is imaging ordered?' therefore is: 'When additional information is necessary to change the management of the patient or outcome of the disease'. Specifically:

(1) confirming/excluding the initial diagnosis;

(2) staging of the disease;

(3) planning management—medical or surgical;

(4) assessing the response to treatment;

(5) demonstrating complications of disease or management;

(6) monitoring for relapse.

But the information needs to be useful or we are wasting our time and doing some harm. Whether the *information* is useful depends on the request by the referring clinician, why the test was ordered, and when it was ordered, as well as on the quality of the information generated in the imaging department and how quickly the information was transferred to the clinician.

Let's update the definition to: to provide *efficacious* imaging that gives information to the referring clinician, *allowing alteration in the management or outcome of the disease* in the shortest time.

## Treatment

If the action threshold has been passed, treatment can proceed.

The nature and extent of the disease is understood. At this stage, you will have to make a decision about *what to do for the best*. Allowance has to be made for:

• the wishes and values of those affected, principally the patient;

• the various possible outcomes;

- the likelihood and risk of each outcome;
- what is hoped for (the importance of each outcome to the patient);
- what is possible (given the severity and extent of the disease, the state of the other organ systems, and the resources available at the time) (Cox 1992).

## Ordering another test

If there is *not enough information*, think about ordering another pathology or imaging test. But spare a moment to think about *what variables to consider when ordering investigations*:

(1) will either a positive or negative result alter the management of the disease or the outcome for the patient;

(2) how long will it take;

(3) the cost;

(4) the radiation to the patient;

(5) the mortality and morbidity.

At last, the definition of the *role of radiology* is shaping up. It would go something like this:

to provide efficacious imaging which gives *information* to the referring clinician allowing alteration of the management of the patient or the outcome of the disease and to provide image-guided therapy, in the shortest time and with the least cost, morbidity, and mortality.

Radiology is not about making the diagnosis at all costs. Mentally, this is an easier pathway but it is expensive for the community and suboptimal for the patient. Like a chess game it is better when one thinks two steps ahead, not to *what is the diagnosis* but to *can this test give information that will alter the management?*

If the test is necessary, it is ordered. The next step is to interpret it.

Most radiology examinations come back to the referring doctor with a report. Sometimes the simpler radiographs do not. A clinician needs to be able to interpret the basic radiographs and, in the more complex studies, correlate the report with the images and the clinical picture.

With plain X-rays, you must do one of three things:

1. Call the film normal.

2. Call it abnormal.

3. If undecided, know when and where to seek help. Help is available from a peer, a superior, a radiologist, and Burgener and Kormano's book *Differential diagnosis in conventional radiology* (1997) or Keats'(1996) *Atlas of normal variants that may simulate disease.*

## What does it mean if the test is normal?

Calling a film normal is often harder than seeing an abnormality. If a CXR with a large opacity is shown it takes one nanosecond to call it abnormal. To call a CXR normal can take a minute or two. Section 1 of this book provides a scheme for viewing radiographs, which combines the viewing of important areas with a logical perceptual flow. A film cannot be called normal until each section has been checked. This system should decrease uncertainty and make life easier.

Seeing a normal film is not time wasted, it is an important educational experience. It adds to the mental databank subtle variations such as a bigger heart in children, larger lungs in older people, and it makes the interpretation of the next film that much easier.

A normal X-ray may effectively exclude disease, moving the probability to below the exclusion threshold.

A note of caution. If an X-ray is normal, it does not always exclude disease. For example, a normal bone X-ray will not exclude osteomyelitis. A normal CXR will not exclude metastatic deposits entirely. How sure do you want to be? Involved lymph nodes could be hidden in the mediastinum and there may be nodules in the lungs that are not visible. A CT could be performed. It is a more sensitive test.

Even a CT, however, has its limitations. Nodes below 1 cm in size are called normal. They are probably not involved, but they could be. There is always some uncertainty, always will be. One of the skills of clinicians is to live with the uncertainty and feel comfortable making a decision about what to do for the best.

> ### Hint
> Sensitivity means the ability of a test to detect disease when it is present. If 100 people have the disease and 80 give an abnormal test, the test has a sensitivity of 80%.

## What does it mean if the test is abnormal?

The abnormality is often obvious; but even so, a systematic approach is needed to search for clues as to its nature and to find a possible second lesion. It takes a long time to become familiar with radiology images. A degree of pattern recognition will develop. However, there is no short cut to looking systematically at every film.

Once the abnormality is found:

1. Describe it. Be on the lookout for good descriptors in radiology reports and add them to your vocabulary.

2. Compare it with previous studies.

3. Classify it with a generic diagnosis: a mass, consolidation, effusion.

4. Give a specific diagnosis only if you are sure.

## What is the significance of the abnormality?

It depends on whether it is a pertinent or incidental finding. A pertinent finding is important. An incidental finding is less important. Any diagnosis becomes more likely if the X-ray appearances agree with the clinical findings.

A pertinent finding such as lobar pneumonia on a CXR will move the probability above the action threshold. In another case, finding a nodule on a CXR will move the probability towards—but not past—the action threshold. Further tests may be needed, such as a CT to clarify the anatomy of the lungs, mediastinum, and liver and a fine-needle biopsy to reveal the nature of the lesion.

## How to avoid errors in interpretation

Errors in interpretation of images occur from three causes:

(1)  technical factors;

(2)  observer performance (search, recognition, decision):

- scanning errors—not seen
- recognition errors—seen but not recognized
- decision-making errors—recognized but with incorrect interpretation;

(3)  lesion characteristics (site, size, shape, conspicuousness).

Following the guidelines in this book will minimize errors for the following reasons:

- Making a decision about 'what to confirm, exclude, define, or show the progress of' before ordering the test will minimize technical errors; a decision on whether to accept the test if negative should have already been decided. A high pretest probability will mean that a negative test (perhaps because of technical factors) does not exclude disease to your satisfaction and another test may be ordered.

- The correct modality will more likely be chosen.

- Using a systematic approach builds experience in the enormous range of what can be normal, and decreases scanning and recognition errors because every image is searched systematically. It is simply a matter of more practice.

- The three-part recognition technique for looking at images should increase detection of lesions of varying site, size, shape, and conspicuousness.

No one is perfect. Even if you are looking for a known pattern or shape it is possible to look at it, or within a millimetre of it, and not recognize it. Take this simple test: how many 'F's are in the following sentence?

> FINISHED FILES ARE THE RE-
> SULT OF YEARS OF SCIEN-
> TIFIC STUDY COMBINED WITH
> THE EXPERIENCE OF YEARS

An answer of three is only half-right, but is what most people see. Missing a finding in an X-ray is therefore unfortunate but entirely understandable. If someone shows you a radiograph that you misinterpret, the correct response is not 'how stupid I am' or even 'how did I miss that?' but rather 'what a great educational case!'

Accept that the mind interprets images in different ways and it takes time and experience to become good at medical imaging. Chest X-rays may seem like a barely organized grouping of dark and light areas at first. With practice, patterns will emerge, like this bust of a bearded man. (Meyers 1995)

If the test result does not show what you thought it should, you have a problem. Is the error in the clinical thinking, in interpretation of the image, or is the disease present and not visible (a false-negative)?

For example: a fall on an outstretched hand. Examination detects tenderness over the scaphoid. Provisional diagnosis is a fracture. Order an X-ray to confirm a

**Fig. 15.5** Bust of a bearded man.

fracture of the scaphoid. The X-ray appears normal. Ask for another opinion if there is a problem in interpretation of the image. You still think it is broken, the disease is present but not visible. Adopt the appropriate risk-management pathway:

- take another view;
- or order another test (CT or radionuclear scan);
- or treat as if present, immobilize it and X-ray again in 10 days;
- or speak to a radiologist about your problem

'Misses' will always occur. It is unfair to call them mistakes. Everyone has them. They are learning opportunities. If it is not a deliberate and malicious error, it is defendable. Misinterpretation rates for radiologists are around 5% and for resident medical staff quite a bit more (Siegle *et al.* 1998) (Tudor *et al.* 1997).

Protection from lawsuits does not lie in ordering more investigations but in the *history*: making the diagnosis from the story, putting it in the context of the person's lifestyle, and establishing a rapport so that a partnership is established and the treatment will be followed. If in retrospect the wrong diagnosis has been decided, or the wrong treatment given, you may find that people can be surprisingly forgiving. If your treatment seemed reasonable at the time and was well documented your defences are well manned and should be difficult to breach.

Follow up patients to find out how they are. Both parties will benefit. Recognizing a gap between your clinical assessment and the eventual diagnosis is an important insight. If there is too much of a gap occurring too often, take some remedial action:

- learn the 200 single-sentence definitions of diseases;
- slow down;
- enrol in some post-graduate education.

More detailed knowledge about each imaging modality would include the following. Some of these details need only be known by a specialist.

- What disease can the test confirm or exclude?
- What anatomy, function, or pathology can it define?
- What is the possibility that it may add further information, given the clinical information and other imaging to date?
- How do you correlate the findings with other imaging?
- How frequently should it be performed to follow progress?
- Will it influence management?
- What is the sensitivity and specificity?
- What is the morbidity and mortality?
- What is its availability?
- What is the cost?
- What do you do next if the test is positive?
- What do you do next if the test is negative?
- What preparation is needed?
- What aftercare is needed?
- How do you explain the findings to the doctor?
- How do you explain the findings to the patient?

## How a radiologist can help

He or she can:

- advise on which test is appropriate;
- perform interventional work;
- report on most examinations;
- correlate complex imaging information from various modalities;
- communicate promptly—leave your telephone number and pager number for better service.

## Probabilities

Now a word or two (about 500 actually) about probability. Sadly, there is only a 50% chance that you will read this section and only an 84% chance that you will understand it.

These paragraphs would be unnecessary if radiology tests were always correct. They are not because:

- the disease is often not visible in the early stages or the late stages;
- some diseases may not be visible at any stage; and
- errors of interpretation do occur.

The test will only detect the disease in a certain percentage of people who have it. Let us say that 80% of people with pneumonia will have an abnormal CXR (a positive result). The sensitivity of the CXR in pneumonia is 80%.

Additionally, the test will be abnormal in a few people who do not have the disease. The test is not 100% specific for the disease. Let us say it has a specificity of 90%, that is 90% of people without the disease will have a normal CXR. If the test was completely specific for the disease, all people without pneumonia would have a normal test; i.e. no false-positives.

Sensitivity means how well the test can detect an abnormality.

Specificity means how well the test can detect normality.

These concepts are important because they allow understanding of the uncertainty of medicine and because a knowledge of sensitivity and specificity is a prerequisite for interpreting many journal articles.

After the history taking and examination if there is a 50/50 chance of pneumonia and then a CXR is performed the probabilities will look like Fig. 15.6:

If the CXR is positive there is an 89% (40/45) chance of pneumonia, up from 50%. If it is negative, there is still an 18% (10/55) chance of pneumonia being present.

Look what happens if the disease was thought to be unlikely, following the information from the history and examination, say only a 10% chance of its presence. The 2 × 2 table would look like Fig. 15.7:

If the CXR is *abnormal*, it is as likely to be a false-positive (9) as it is a true-positive (8). That could be a bit confusing.

Look at the situation where at the end of the history and examination pneumonia is considered highly likely, say 90% sure. The 2 × 2 table will be as in Fig. 15.8.

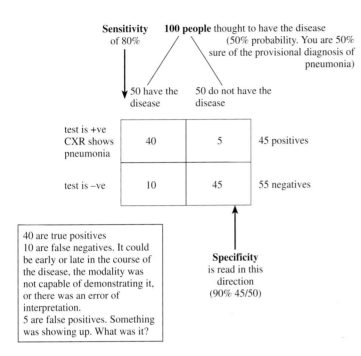

**Fig. 15.6** What does it mean if the test is positive or negative?

Sensitivity of 80%

**100 people** thought to have the disease (50% probability. You are 50% sure of the provisional diagnosis of pneumonia)

50 have the disease

50 do not have the disease

| | 50 have the disease | 50 do not have the disease | |
|---|---|---|---|
| test is +ve CXR shows pneumonia | 40 | 5 | 45 positives |
| test is –ve | 10 | 45 | 55 negatives |

40 are true positives
10 are false negatives. It could be early or late in the course of the disease, the modality was not capable of demonstrating it, or there was an error of interpretation.
5 are false positives. Something was showing up. What was it?

**Specificity** is read in this direction (90% 45/50)

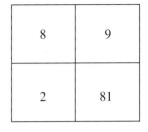

| 8 | 9 |
|---|---|
| 2 | 81 |

**Fig. 15.7** With an estimated 10% chance of disease before the test was ordered.

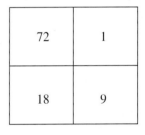

| 72 | 1 |
|---|---|
| 18 | 9 |

**Fig. 15.8** With an estimated 90% chance of disease before the test was ordered.

If 100 people have similar signs and symptoms, 90 will have pneumonia. The CXR will identify 72 (80%) of these. A total of 73 will appear to have pneumonia on the X-ray. If the test is positive, certainty has increased from 90% to 99%. Was it worth doing the test? Of the 27 people who appear to have a normal CXR, many have the disease but it is not visible, or not recognized. In fact, there are more false negatives than true negatives.

It is not possible to detail the reliability, limitations, dangers, and costs of different investigations because of so much local variation. It becomes intuitive after a while. If in doubt, consult a friendly radiologist.

## To put radiology in perspective...

Sometimes the medical course feels like a motoring trip through Europe without a map. You come to Vaduz in Liechtenstein where a guide skilfully and correctly explains the locality and sends you on the road to Venice. You would like to know where you are, where you have been, where you are going, and how it all fits together in the grand scheme. Here is the map.

The medical school teaches:

(1) basic science: anatomy, physiology, biochemistry, microbiology, *et al.*;

(2) diagnosis, clinical judgement, and management of diseases which can be classified by the international classification of diseases (ICD) or by the principal types of pathological change:

- congenital and genetic
- physical
- chemical, biochemical, toxic, and metabolic
- inflammatory, allergic, and immunological
- neoplastic and cystic
- nutritional
- functional
- psychiatric
- changes secondary to changes in other organs and systems
- unknown;

(3)  personal development:

- acquiring skills in communication, treatment procedures, problem solving, the scientific method, ethics, self-appraisal, self-motivation, enthusiasm, self-confidence, and commitment;

(4)  group and community issues:

- knowledge of the healthcare system, prevention of disease, and teamwork.

Medical imaging is an important but not a big player. It adds information in many, but not all, of the disease processes in category 2.

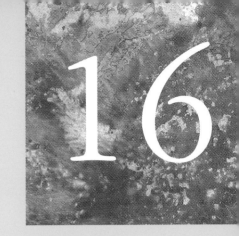

# 16

# *Understanding imaging modalities*

- MRI
- Ultrasound
- CT
- Radionuclear imaging
- Key concepts in medical imaging
  *CXR*
  *AXR*
  *Facial bones*
  *Cervical spine*
  *Orthopaedics*
  *CT head*
  *History taking*
  *Clinical thinking*

- Finally

## Cervical spine

Check that it is the correct film and then look at the:

*Lateral view*:

- the body of T1 should be visible,
- start at the front, the prevertebral tissues, and look up and down the structures from anterior to posterior until reaching the spinous processes;

*AP view*:

- spinous processes, vertebral bodies, intervertebral discs, lateral masses;

*Peg view*:

- odontoid peg
- alignment of C1–C2.

## Orthopaedics

Check that it is the correct film and then look at the:

(1)  medulla and cortex of the bones

(2)  joint spaces and alignment

(3)  soft tissues

## CT head

Check that it is the correct film and then look at the:

(1)  ventricles—are they normal in site, size, and configuration?

(2)  cerebral and cerebellar attenuation

(3)  skull, sinuses, orbits, and facial bones.

(4)  is there any space-occupying lesion or haemorrhage within the cranial cavity or any abnormality outside the cranial cavity?

## History taking

There are three features.

1. If possible, come up with a *provisional diagnosis* (hypothesis) so that the examination, and subsequent investigations if any, will be directed to confirm, exclude, define, or show the progress of the diagnosis.

2. Put the *disease in the context of the patient's lifestyle* and use clinical judgement to relate the probability of the diagnosis to what can reasonably be achieved, considering the age, prior and concurrent illnesses, effect of the illness, and the expectations of the patient.

3. *Establish a relationship with the patient*, a mutual trust that allows understanding of the diagnosis, the treatment, and the uncertainties and complications that may occur. A recipe for success.

## Clinical thinking

In cases where the diagnosis is not apparent from the history, or the history plus examination, or when more information is needed, consider the following questions.

1. What is the working diagnosis or differential diagnosis?
2. What do I need to know?
3. Which imaging modality or pathology test will confirm, exclude, define, or show the progress of this?
4. What may be shown, and where do I go from here?

## Finally

Read the preface before reading the book for a second time. Better not to hurry. Remember that understanding, like friendship, takes time to develop.

If you have any questions or suggestions, please send me an e-mail at *p.scally@mailbox.uq.edu.au* or fax +61 7 3840 1850.

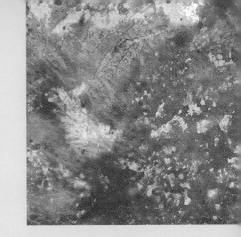

# Further reading

# Further reading

Barrows, H.S. and Pickell, G.C. (1991). *Developing clinical problem-solving skills, a guide to more effective diagnosis and treatment.* Norton Medical, New York. (*A useful guide to clinical thinking and decision-making processes. The 220 pages may seem daunting but this is a critical skill to be mastered. The book will lead to a net saving of time and better patient care.*)

Chapman, S. and Nakielny, R. (1995). *Aids to radiological differential diagnosis* (3rd edn). W.B. Saunders, London. (*More a book for radiology trainees. Great lists of differentials.*)

Cotran, R.S., Kumar, V., and Robbins, S.L. (1994). *Pathologic basis of disease* (5th edn). W.B. Saunders, Philadelphia. (*An essential reference. Unfortunately studied too early in the medical course in many instances to have its proper impact. Worth revisiting.*)

Daffner, R.H. (1993). *Clinical radiology, the essentials.* Williams and Wilkins, Baltimore, MD. (*Another approach to radiology teaching.*)

Grainger, R.G. and Allison, D. (1997) Diagnostic Radiology: A textbook of medical imaging (3rd edn). Churchill Livingstone, New York. (*Available in most medical imaging departments and libraries. A first class reference for information about areas of interest.*)

Greenspan, A. (1996). *Orthopedic radiology* (2nd edn). Lippincott-Raven, Philadelphia. (*Beautifully displayed reference for those who would like to be more familiar with orthopedic radiology.*)

Hope, R.A., Longmore, J.M., McManus, S.K., and Wood-Allum, C.A. (1998). *Oxford handbook of clinical medicine* (4th edn). Oxford University Press. (*Very useful handbook for students and doctors.*)

Keats, T.E. and Smith, T.H. (1988). *An atlas of normal developmental roentgen anatomy* (2nd edn). Year Book Medical Publishers Inc., Chicago. (*An essential reference for when confronted with young bones and shapes that are unfamiliar.*)

Kumar, P.J. (1998). *Clinical medicine* (4th edn). W.B. Saunders, London. (*Comprehensive coverage of clinical medicine.*)

Lau, L. (ed.) (1997). *Imaging guidelines* (3rd edn.). Royal Australasian College of Radiologists and Victorian Medical Postgraduate Foundation Inc., 293 Royal Parade, Parkville, Victoria, Australia. fax +61 3 9347 4547. (*An inexpensive book that gives pathways/algorithms for investigating common clinical problems. Can be useful as a reference for general practitioners.*)

Raby, N., Berman, L., and de Lacey, G. (1995). *Accident and emergency radiology, a survival guide.* W.B. Saunders, London. (*This book is a classic in its presentation and understanding of the basic radiology that needs to be known by emergency department personnel.*)

RCR. (1995). *Making the best use of a Department of Clinical Radiology, guidelines for doctors* (3rd edn). The guidelines secretary, RCR, 38 Portland Place, London W1N 4JQ. (*This little guide contains valuable advice of what to order and when. It will save you time, save the health provider money, and spare the patient some exposure to radiation.*)

W.B. Saunders (1994). *Dorland's illustrated medical dictionary* (28th edn). W.B. Saunders, Philadelphia. (*Like all dictionaries, this one should be consulted more often.*)

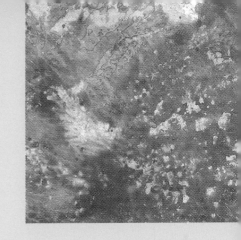

References

# References

Abboud, P-A.C., Malet, P.F., Berlin, J.A., *et al*. (1996). Predictors of common bile duct stones prior to cholecystectomy: a meta-analysis. *Gastrointestinal Endoscopy*, 44, 450–9.

Burgener, F.A. and Kormano, M. (1991). *Differential diagnosis in conventional radiology* (2nd edn). Thième, Stuttgart.

Chapman, S. and Nakielny, R. (1995). *Aids to radiological differential diagnosis* (3rd edn), pp. 569–71. W.B. Saunders, London.

Cox, K. (1992). What doctors need to know. A note on professional performance. *Medical Journal of Australia*, 157, 764–8.

Dolan, D.D. and Jacoby, C.G. (1978). Facial fractures. *Seminars in Roentgenology*, 13, 37.

Greenspan, A. (1996). *Orthopedic radiology* (2nd edn). Lippincott–Raven, Philadelphia.

Hall, F.M. (1996). Viewing mammograms. *American Journal of Roentgenology*, 166, 465. (Letter)

Hardison, J.E. (1979). To be complete. *New England Journal of Medicine*, 300, 193–4.

Helms, C.A. (1989). *Fundamentals of skeletal radiology* (2nd edn), p. 1. W.B. Saunders, Philadelphia.

Keats, T.E. (1996). *Atlas of normal roentgen variants that may simulate disease* (6th edn). Mosby Year Book, St Louis.

Keats, T.E. and Smith, T.H. (1988). *An atlas of normal developmental roentgen anatomy* (2nd edn). Year Book Medical Publishers, Chicago.

Lloyd, D.A., Carty, H., Patterson, M., Roe, D. and Butcher, C.K. (1997). Predictive value of skull radiography for intracranial injury in children with blunt head injury. *Lancet*, 349, 821–4.

McMahon, P., Grossman, W., Gaffney, M., and Stanitski, C. (1995). Soft-tissue injury as an indication of child abuse. *Journal of Bone and Joint Surgery* (American volume) 77, 1179–83.

Marzano, R. (1992). *A different kind of classroom*. Association for supervision and curriculum, Alexandria, VA.

Meyers, M.A. (1995). Science, creativity, and serendipity. *American Journal of Roentgenology*, 165, 755–64.

Mohler, S.R. (1996). Flight crews and cabin crews encouraged to increase awareness of in-flight ionising radiation. Human factors and aviation medicine. *Flight Safety Foundation*, 23, 1–4.

Raby, N., Berman, L., and de Lacey, G. (1995). *Accident and emergency radiology, a survival guide*. W.B. Saunders, London.

RCR (1995). Making the best use of a Department of Clinical Radiology, guidelines for doctors (3rd edn). The Royal College of Radiologists, London.

Siegle, R.L., Baram, E.M., Reuter, S.R., Clarke, E.A., Lancaster, J.L., and McMahan, C.A. (1998). Rates of disagreement in imaging interpretation in a group of community hospitals. *Academic Radiology*, 5, 148–54.

Tudor, G.R., Finlay, D., and Taub, N. (1997). An assessment of inter-observer agreement and accuracy when reporting plain radiographs. *Clinical Radiology*, 52, 235–8.

Van der Jagt, E. and Smits, H.J. (1992). Cardiac size in the supine chest film. *European Journal of Radiology*, 14, 173–7.

Verma, S., Hamilton, K., Hawkins, H.H., Kothari, R., Singal, B., Buncher, R., Nguyen, P., and O'Neill, M. (1997). Clinical application of the Ottawa ankle rules for the use of radiography in acute ankle injuries. *American Journal of Roentgenology*, 169, 825–7.

Weber, B.G. (1972). *Die Verletzungen des Oberen Sprunggelenkes*. Verlag Hans Huber, Stuttgart.

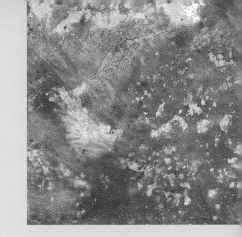

# Index

Page numbers in *italics* refer to figures